OF MICE, MEN, AND MICROBES
Hantavirus

OF MICE, MEN, AND MICROBES

Hantavirus

David R. Harper

Andrea S. Meyer

Academic Press

San Diego London Boston New York Sydney Tokyo Toronto

Academic Press
a division of Harcourt Brace & Company
525 B Street, Suite 1900, San Diego, California 92101-4495, USA
http://www.apnet.com

Academic Press
24-28 Oval Road, London NW1 7DX, UK
http://www.hbuk.co.uk/ap/

Library of Congress Catalog Card Number: 99-60590

International Standard Book Number: 0-12-326460-X

PRINTED IN THE UNITED STATES OF AMERICA
99 00 01 02 03 04 MM 9 8 7 6 5 4 3 2 1

This book is dedicated to our children.

CONTENTS

FOREWORD ix
ACKNOWLEDGMENTS xiii

1 THE HEART OF AMERICA/THE MIDDLE OF
   NOWHERE 1

2 AN OUTBREAK OF FEAR 13

3 UNRAVELING THE MYSTERY 27

4 PUTTING THE PUZZLE TOGETHER 41

5 OF MICE AND MEN 59

6 AT LAST, A PLAN 79

7 HANTAVIRUSES: OUT OF ASIA 99

8   OTHER HANTAVIRUSES 117

9   THREE BILLION YEARS 131

10   ON THE ORIGIN OF VIRUSES 145

11   CHANGES, CONCEALMENT, AND
     TROJAN HORSES 163

12   COUSINS 183

13   WHAT WE KNOW 199

14   HOW TO STOP A VIRUS 215

15   OUTBREAKS 233

     APPENDIX A: Centers for Disease Control Guidelines
                  on Prevention of HPS 249
     APPENDIX B: Sources of Further Information 257
     APPENDIX C: Abbreviations 265
     INDEX 267

FOREWORD
. . . .

IF IT CAN HAPPEN HERE . . .

As part of the most scientifically advanced society in the history of mankind, we Americans often feel distanced and insulated, perhaps even immune, from the disease epidemics that ravage many parts of the "undeveloped" world. Medical science has beaten the historic scourges of our culture—smallpox, cholera, bubonic plague, polio—and is rapidly closing on many others. Childhood vaccination programs in the United States have so reduced many common diseases that an occasional small cluster of cases is cause for public alarm. Americans traveling overseas must still "get their shots" before leaving home, unlike visitors coming to the United States; North America is perceived as a microbially benign environment. Even the introduction of AIDS to the United States did not panic our population. Viewed widely as a "lifestyle" disease, generally acquired through voluntary behaviors and easily avoided with appropriate precautions, AIDS did not pack the sheer horror of historic epidemics; it lacked the mystery, the apparent randomness, of diseases that can spread quickly, relentlessly, and mercilessly to all quarters of society. Despite the masses of casualties and the horrendous cost in lives and resources, AIDS did not terrorize the American populace.

Many in America seem to have forgotten, or never knew, the history of disease epidemics in the United States. Foremost among the 20th century pandemics was the 1918 influenza ("Spanish Flu") which swept across the country, killing tens of thousands of Americans in only four months. Transported to Europe in the late summer by American "doughboys" heading for the trenches of World War I, the influenza circled the globe and claimed the lives of more than 20 million victims. Nearly 1% of the entire world's population was killed by this virus in less than a year. Today, only our elders can recall the events, and our society's collective memory of the epidemic is being relegated to the history books. Ancient history. From a scientifically primitive America. Can't happen again. Not here. Not now.

But just when we believed our scientific prowess could justify our confidence, Nature shattered the illusion. In the spring of 1993, the American Southwest suffered an outbreak of an unknown, deadly disease that displayed many of the hallmarks of a terrible plague—mysterious origins, apparently random victims, agonizing pain, rapid death, no treatment, no cure. What was it? Where did it come from? How do you fight it? Why here? Why now?

David Harper and Andrea Meyer have put together a riveting account of the events of that period, describing the events leading up to the Sin Nombre hantavirus outbreak and following the story through the summer of 1998. As a team, they have brought to bear their expertise in medical science and the Southwestern culture to provide a clear and insightful picture of the complex events of 1993. With a presentation style of short, direct essays on individual aspects, the story flows seamlessly through the stages of the outbreak, linking together the myriad activities of medical personnel, scientists, field biologists, the news media, and the American populace. The resulting account provides both a history of the events and an explanation for those events—the "whys" and "wherefores" that often are glossed over in the short sound bytes of modern media coverage.

But the story is not confined solely to the Sin Nombre hantavirus. David Harper is a virologist by training, and he brings to the book a vast knowledge of virus biology and genetics. In clear and nontechnical presentations, he explains the workings of viruses in their hosts (or victims), describing how viruses gain entry to the cells, what they do to cause disease, and how our immune system is mobilized to the defense. But viruses are moving targets, changing their genetic make-up to thwart the defenses; thus, Dr. Harper describes the evolution of the genetic "arms race" between virus and host, a continual maneuvering by each entity to gain the upper hand in the battle for survival. Finally, in addition to the outbreak's history, the authors have compiled a compendium of hantavirus information, including references on viruses, details of the CDC-recommended methods for preventing hantaviral diseases, and a listing of Internet addresses for hantavirus-related homepages.

Of Mice, Men, and Microbes provides a scientifically accurate and critical appraisal of a disease outbreak, and this book will serve not only as a history of the events but also as a forewarning of things to come. The Sin Nombre hantavirus outbreak has taught us yet again that history will repeat itself and that disease epidemics are the rule rather than the exception. It did happen here. And it will again.

Dr. Robert R. Parmenter
Albuquerque, New Mexico

ACKNOWLEDGMENTS

Many of the illustrations in this book were taken, with permission, from the Centers for Disease Control Hantavirus information web pages. Illustrations from this source were photographs of the deer mouse, white-footed mouse, cotton rat, and rice rat; electron micrograph of the Sin Nombre virus; case map for hantavirus pulmonary syndrome since 1994; and a map of probable effects of El Niño on rainfall. In addition, maps of hantavirus pulmonary syndrome cases by state and of the distributions of the deer mouse, white-footed mouse, cotton rat, and rice rat were based on maps from this site combined with information from other sources. These illustrations are used courtesy of Special Pathogens Branch, Division of Viral and Rickettsial Diseases, National Center for Infectious Diseases, and Centers for Disease Control and Prevention.

The photograph of a worker at the Sevilleta quarantine site was taken by Dr. Brian Hjelle, University of New Mexico, and is used with his permission. The map of the Sevilleta site is derived from maps from the Sevilleta long-term ecological research program website and is used with permission from Dr.

Robert Parmenter, University of New Mexico and Sevilleta LTER Program. The photograph of the Dolores Canyon is used courtesy of Gail Binkly. The photographs of rodent surveys "before and after" were provided by Dr. Terry Yates, University of New Mexico, and are used with his permission.

Quotations concerning the El Bolson Argentinian hantavirus outbreak are taken from the Health I.G. Consultora Periodística hantavirus information website, with permission.

The authors thank the many people who have given freely of their time during the preparation of this book, without whose cooperation it would not have been possible. The authors thank Charles Calisher, Jim Cheek, John DeWitt, Natalie Dolan, Dennis Garrison, Diane Goade, Brian Hjelle, Andrew Hope, Marla Jasperse, Fred Koster, Marc Meyer, Stuart Nichol, John Pape, Bob Parmenter, Cheryl Parmenter, Carol Percy, Chris Percy, C. J. Peters, Connie Schmaljohn, and Bruce Tempest. We thank, especially, those patients and their families who spoke about their experiences. In addition, we thank the organizers of the Fourth International Conference on HFRS and Hantaviruses, held in Atlanta, Georgia, March 1998. We also thank those news organizations that opened their files to our research.

We thank Tessa Picknett at Harcourt Brace publishers, who gave us the judicious mixture of rein and support we needed during the writing of this book.

I, Andrea Meyer, thank all the friends who loaned me books and ideas and who helped to focus my thoughts. Thanks go as well to my colleagues at Cortez Newspapers, who are also my friends, and who have been supportive throughout this project. Special appreciation goes to my husband, Marc, and my children, Jacob and Katie, who gave freely of their time so that my own time was free to write this book and who have served, since the very beginning, as a test market for my words. Bless you, kids, for believing in me and for cooking our dinner.

I, David Harper, thank colleagues, friends, and family for time, support, and coffee, as well as St. Bartholomew's and the Royal London Medical and Dental School, within Queen Mary and Westfield College (University of London), for providing sabbatical leave at critical times.

Our internet service providers and Mirabilis Ltd. deserve gratitude as well. Without that technology the process of collaborating across the Atlantic and half a continent would have been slow and frustrating, rather than just frustrating.

THE HEART OF AMERICA/ THE MIDDLE OF NOWHERE

· ·

The insufferable arrogance of human beings to think that Nature was made solely for their benefit, as if it was conceivable that the sun had been set afire merely to ripen men's apples and head their cabbages.

SAVINIEN CYRANO DE BERGERAC,
L'Histoire comique des etats et empires de la lune

· ·

The high desert of the American southwest does not surrender its secrets easily.

This is a place where change is marked in natural rhythms rather than on any human calendar, and sometimes only the broadest cycles—the eons, the epochs—are visible to the casual observer. The forces of change are sometimes as big as all outdoors—scorching sun, inexorable wind, and torrents of water aided and abetted by gravity. They are not invisible, exactly, but they are most often unseen. The very rocks themselves, in hues that are brilliant and at the same time subtle, stand in mute testimony to the powers that have created and continue to define this place. One only has to look carefully.

To visitors, the high desert seems empty. It is not; indeed, it is richly inhabited. The scale is simply so vast that it does not initially encourage close inspection, instead drawing the eye to sweeping vistas and the intellect to equally sweeping generalizations. Such perspectives miss a great deal.

Other rhythms add life to this seemingly timeless place. A desert may have been the inspiration for the phrase, "as different as day from night," because the nocturnal face is much different, much busier, than the one it turns to the harsh rays of the sun. Beyond the circadian rhythms, there are those of the seasons: the frozen silence of winter, springtimes of riotous rebirth, broiling summers, and then the frenzy of preparation that is autumn. Beyond even those are the longer and less predictable cycles of drought and flood, of feast and famine. Lately, humans have added their own twists: invasion and exodus, boom and bust.

This is also a place of interfaces. Some are as apparent as the contrast of red sandstone and blue sky at the horizon, whereas some will probably never be made known to humans. On a map of the southwest, state boundaries converge at a place called, prosaically enough, "The Four Corners." Colorado, New Mexico, Arizona, and Utah meet at a common point, the only point in the United States where four states meet. Ironically, those state boundaries are largely irrelevant because superimposed on them are the boundaries of other political entities, the sovereign Native American nations whose laws take precedence within the reservation boundaries. Underlying those arbitrary lines are physical features wrought by forces far more enduring than human doctrine. There are mountains that send water flowing to oceans on either side of a great continent. There are canyons, carrying that water, that are impossible to cross. Those geographic realities create another interface, that between man and nature, and along that margin there is constant conflict.

In 1993, when residents of the Four Corners began to die of an unfamiliar disease, all these outlines became important, for many different reasons.

WHY HERE? WHY NOW?

The arid landscape defines all that happens there. Humans have attempted to live in the Four Corners for millennia; some have adapted to the realities of desert life, but many more have passed from the picture. Grand Canyon explorer John Wesley Powell, who was an ethnographer as well as an adventurer, wrote that water would be the limiting factor in the settlement of those parts of the North American continent lying west of the 100th meridian (which runs through the Dakotas, Nebraska, Kansas, Oklahoma, and Texas, all of them one tier east of the Four Corners states). Powell based that opinion on his observations of not only the flora and fauna of the Colorado plateau but of its human inhabitants as well. His intent was to urge judicious use of a finite resource, not to start a water grab, but perhaps the most convincing proof that he was right was the damming of the Colorado River to construct namesake Lake Powell, a huge reservoir that now supplies water to the cities of the West.

As Powell observed, the West is a dry place with a long past. Streams that are trickles most of the year and torrents for a few months each spring arch against canyon walls, unable to under-cut but unwilling just to slip on past. Every year millions of visitors stand on the rim of the Grand Canyon, amazed that such a chasm could have been eroded one grain of sand at a time, their minds unable to encompass the notion that time has plodded along for so many millions of years before humans arrived to supervise it.

Faded gray-green plants such as sage and rabbitbrush and pygmy trees such as juniper and piñons have long lives and imperceptible growth patterns. Their very lack of lushness al-lows them to survive in a landscape characterized by unfiltered sun and little moisture. They have lessons to teach about the effective use of available resources.

The animal denizens of the desert are generally discreet. Some live their entire lives underground. Many are nocturnal. Most, from the smallest reptiles to the largest carnivores, are well camouflaged. A sharp eye detects that the birds soaring on the thermals are mostly raptors and scavengers; there are song-birds in this place, but they too do not advertise themselves too loudly.

The Native Americans to whom much of this land belongs are reverent to what outsiders consider to be the mysteries of life. Completely embedded in the interior of the most highly developed country on earth, the Navajo homeland is a sover-eign nation with a strong identity of its own. Like the very colors of the desert, the Navajo way of life hints at strong contrasts, and one of those dichotomies is that in this timeless land, time is in many ways moving very rapidly. The intense blue of the overarching sky is often smudged by emissions from coal-fired power plants in the Four Corners area, plants that provide jobs for Native Americans and income for their tribes while irrevo-cably changing the nature of their home. Litter clutters the roadsides. Some of the most beautiful scenery can now be reached by highways that are paved (although not necessarily smooth; nature does win some of her battles!). Many residents now live in prefabricated housing or in mobile homes—awkward boxes of tin or plywood, perched awkwardly in an environment that tends to round off square corners.

Still, the dominant features of the landscape are those that were here when the first human beings emerged into the blinding sun of this place. Its very openness and the fury of its resident elements seem to have purified it, and many people come here, either as migrants or as pilgrims, in search of that elemental purity.

It is not a scene where an outsider would expect frightening diseases to emerge.

Modern society thinks of diseases as somehow "dirty" rather than as part of any ecosystem, and the southwestern desert does not present itself as unclean. It does not teem with squalling, battling life; this is not a reeking swamp or an open sewer. Indeed, the combination of the daytime sun, winter cold and exposure to light and radiation allowed by its high altitude and clean air make the surface of the desert an inhospitable place for most living things. However, microbes are the first living organisms to colonize a new territory, and from then on, they coexist alongside other forms of life, from the smallest and least complicated to the humans who try so hard to gain dominion over all the earth.

No one here imagines that dominion has been accomplished. Like all living things in the Four Corners, people have the choice of adapting or facing a lifelong struggle. Even at the dawn of the millenium, many of the realities here are extremely physical. The age-old cycle of drought and abundance is never forgotten. AIDS has taken its place as a health threat, but here it must compete for attention with plague. The disease that killed millions in 14th-century Europe is spread here by the fleas hosted by prairie dogs. There are other animal-borne diseases that demand attention, including, occasionally, rabies.

This is still not, by any stretch of the imagination, a human-dominated environment. If a disease were going to emerge here, it would not likely be one that depended on *Homo sapiens* for its survival.

In the spring of 1993, though, a disease did emerge into the public eye, and it set into motion several chains of events that will not soon be forgotten in the Four Corners.

INDEX CASES

In mid-May 1993, when rumors of a "mystery disease" began circulating throughout the Four Corners area of the southwestern United States, details were sparse and often contradictory. The most striking aspect of the story was that the first identified victim had been young and healthy. A long-distance runner, 19-year-old Merrill Bahe certainly did not fit the profile of the population group most likely to die from a respiratory illness. We know from influenza, pneumonia, and the many other diseases that target the lungs that typical victims are the very young, the very old, and the unwell. Merrill Bahe was none of these.

He grew up on the very edge of the Navajo reservation, an outstanding athlete and later a track star at Santa Fe Indian School, where he met Florena Woody, another student athlete. In April 1993, the couple was living with their young son in a trailer in the Woody family compound at Littlewater, New Mexico. While it was Merrill Bahe who brought the attention of the world to the Four Corners, he was not the first in his family to develop the new and terrifying illness.

On April 29, 1993, Florena Woody experienced aching muscles. A few days later, she developed a fever and the symptoms of flu. As these worsened, she was admitted to the nearby Crownpoint Hospital on May 8. The next day, she was suffering from massive pneumonia and deep shock. X-rays showed that her lungs were filling with fluid. She was given oxygen while awaiting transfer to an intensive care unit, but all that could be done was not enough. Florena Woody died on Mother's Day, May 9, 1993.

Merrill Bahe had also developed a flu-like illness. On May 11, he visited Crownpoint Hospital, where the doctors were concerned because he had the same symptoms. He was given various medications in an attempt to control the unidentified illness, including Tylenol for the discomfort, antibiotics to target bacterial respiratory infection, and an antiviral drug used to control influenza, and was sent home. They didn't work.

Three days later he felt so ill he could not attend Florena Woody's funeral in Gallup. His condition had deteriorated so dramatically that family members decided to take him to Gallup anyway, to the large Indian Health Service (IHS) hospital there. The drive is only 60 miles, but the disease progressed so rapidly that he did not survive the trip. Merrill Bahe was pronounced dead on arrival at the Indian Medical Center in Gallup on Friday, May 14.

The attending physician, Dr. Bruce Tempest, had many years of experience working with Native Americans and with the diseases of the American southwest, but this disease was unfamiliar to him. He called the state medical examiner's office, alerting them to a possible problem, and IHS epidemiologist Jim Cheek was also informed.

The state medical examiner, Richard Malone, decided that an autopsy was needed, which requires permission from the victim's family. Requesting such permission was a delicate task. Speaking the name of the recently dead is thought to disturb that person's spirit and risk creating a *chindi,* a ghost. IHS providers, very respectful of traditional religious beliefs about death and the dead, were careful to explain why such a procedure was important.

To the immense relief of the clinicians, Bahe's family gave permission, and they explained why. They told the physicians of Florena Woody's recent death from a similar disease and that, indeed, she was to be buried that day.

That piece of information triggered mental alarms among health-care workers already concerned about an unexplained death. It became quickly apparent that Florena Woody's body should be examined as well, which made it imperative that her burial not take place. Once again, a family was asked a painful question. Once again, they agreed.

THE INVESTIGATION BEGINS

Autopsies were performed on both bodies by University of New Mexico pathologist Dr. Patty McFeeley. She was struck most by the condition of the lungs. Weighing twice what they would normally, and dark bluish-red from lack of oxygen, they were filled with fluid squeezed from the blood. This was very, very surprising in otherwise fit, healthy young people.

By now, the attention of a group of alert clinicians was focused on the case, which was to become the heads-up "index case" for what was to follow.

THE USUAL SUSPECTS

Dr. Tempest studied the records and identified five cases with similar symptoms since late 1992. All were fatal and all involved young Navajos living on the reservation or close to it. All had suffered the same massive flooding of the lungs, an extreme or "fulminant" form of pneumonia. They fitted into the classification of adult respiratory distress syndrome (ARDS). Although ARDS kills tens of thousand of people in the United States each year, it is normally the end stage of another disease or the result of a severe trauma. The majority of ARDS is seen in the elderly. These young, healthy patients were not typical ARDS cases.

Dr. Tempest contacted the New Mexico Department of Health to request tests for possible causes, but what were the suspects?

First: plague, a relatively rare disease that, every so often, emerges to kill.

Plague is a rodent-borne disease, transmitted to humans by the fleas that live on those rodents. In the Southwest, prairie dogs and squirrels are hosts to plague; so are mice. Three forms of plague strike humans: bubonic, pneumonic, and septicemic. The cause of all three is the same: the bacterium *Yersinia pestis*. In many cases, humans are infected when their pets kill plague-bearing rodents and become host to their fleas.

Because the respiratory form of plague begins as a flu-like illness and ends as an overwhelming pneumonia, it was an obvious suspect in the cases of Merrill Bahe and Florena Woody. Although plague is a word usually used in the context of Medieval Europe, in fact the southwestern United States is the largest focus of plague in the world today, with 68 officially reported cases in New Mexico from 1984 to 1994. Some residents say the count is much higher.

When diagnosed early, plague can be treated effectively with antibiotics, but untreated plague kills most of its victims, as many as 75% in bubonic plague and 90% or more in its rarer pneumonic and septicemic manifestations.

Although statistically very rare, plague has a troubling history. In its pneumonic form it can bypass the vector and spread from person to person. Up to 28 million Europeans fell victim to plague in the Middle Ages, over one-third of the population. Plague is still a sizable problem in some areas of the world, and even in developed countries it is handled very carefully because of the awareness of what happened once and might possibly happen again.

That level of contagion and mortality has been reduced drastically by modern medicine, and simple sanitation plays a big part. Plague is a known commodity (and a bacterium, not a virus); it is not likely to ever again pose the threat it did in the Middle Ages. We are now armed with quicker diagnosis, knowledge of the causative agents of disease, and effective treatments

The next killer plague isn't likely to be *Y. pestis,* and this killer wasn't.

New Mexico has one of the best and most experienced plague laboratories in the world. Samples taken by Dr. McFeely were quickly tested, and by Sunday, May 16, it was clear that there were no signs of plague. One of the obvious suspects had been eliminated.

Tests had also been carried out for the most common viral causes of pneumonia, including influenza. The "Spanish" influenza of 1918–1919 killed at least half a million Americans. It was a sudden disease of the respiratory system, killing in hours. There had been a near miss in 1976, when a virus looking very like the Spanish influenza had shown up at Fort Dix, New Jersey. That one did not spread. The fear of a new "Spanish flu" is always with us. The viral studies on these two victims, however, were all negative.

On Monday, May 17, the first investigators arrived at the trailer where Merrill Bahe and Florena Woody had lived. Knowing nothing about what had killed the young couple, they looked around for any likely indicators, without taking any more than normal care. A few days later, Jim Cheek from the IHS also examined the trailer, taking no special precautions against any infection. With plague ruled out, he was considering another possible cause of sudden respiratory distress: poison.

Phosgene is the common name of carbonyl chloride and is a poison gas. Phosgene was first used by the Germans in 1915 on the Western Front, but was quickly adopted by the Allies, accounting for over four-fifths of gas casualties in World War I. Exposure was not instantly fatal, but rather caused the lungs to become hugely inflamed, often killing several days after exposure. Military use of killers like this was outlawed under the Geneva Protocol of 1925, but as usual, there are civilian applications.

A closely related compound, phosphene, is used to control prairie dogs, and exposure to phosphene is also known to be a cause of ARDS. The spring of 1993 was wet and fertile, with rodent numbers increasing throughout the region. To Dr. Cheek, it seemed likely that prairie dog control efforts could have resulted in exposure to phosphene. That was one of the main things he and his team were looking for that day, but he found nothing at all to indicate that phosphene had been used.

Thoroughness is one of the keys to locating the cause of a disease, and Dr. Cheek and his team were thorough. They took blood samples from the family and samples from animals around the trailer. During the examination of the area, they found clear signs that rodents had infested the trailer, but no smoking gun was found, no obvious reason for the deaths of Florena Woody and Merrill Bahe. It was time for more tests.

THE NUMBERS MOUNT

Grief brings families together. On May 11, 2 days after her death, Florena Woody's brother Franklin Woody and his pregnant wife Jackie arrived at the family home. They had come from urban Seattle, moving into the trailer in which Merrill Bahe and Florena Woody had lived. On May 22, Franklin Woody developed a fever and aching muscles. With the events of the recent past very much in mind, he was admitted immediately to the Indian Medical Center at Gallup. Two days later he was transferred to the University of New Mexico (UNM) Medical Center in Albuquerque to be close to intensive care facilities if they were needed. His wife accompanied him.

In Franklin Woody's case, the disease was milder, and the move to Albuquerque may not have been necessary. As it turned out, however, it was very fortunate that he was at UNM, because at that same time, Jackie Woody also started to develop the signs of the new illness. In her case it was a very close call, even with the hugely capable intensive care support she received at UNM. She survived, just, although her child was born at UNM 2 months early and lived only a few months. This did not seem to be due to infection of the unborn child, but her severe illness undoubtedly played a part.

By now, the epidemiologists were very worried indeed. Four young, active individuals living in close proximity were identified as suffering from the new disease. The two later cases had been in contact with Merrill Bahe for 4 days of his illness. An obvious conclusion was that they had been infected from him during that time, which led to the major fear of another epidemic or even the worldwide version, a pandemic. There was a new and unknown infectious disease on the loose, killing half of the people it infected.

The idea that Americans do not die of disease is false. Everyone dies of something, and for those who successfully avoid trauma, the failure of bodily functions from some other cause will eventually kill. That is disease. Americans like to believe that disease culls the weak, the old, the sick. It saddens us, but doesn't alarm us. This disease seemed to be doing the opposite. The most chillingly effective way to destroy a population is to kill off those members who ensure the survival of others, to aim at the heart of that group: healthy, young, vital people.

2

AN OUTBREAK OF FEAR

· · · · · · · · · · · · ·

Knowledge humanizes mankind, and reason inclines to mild-ness; but prejudices destroy every tender disposition.

BARON DE MONTESQUIEU

· ·

Fear is the mind-killer   FRANK HERBERT, *Dune*

· ·

THE SENTINEL

Although suffering from many disadvantages attendant on its existence as an agency of the United States government, the Indian Health Service may have been the ideal agency to identify the problem and respond quickly. Had those initial cases been separated further by either time or distance, or had the physicians not had a framework of communication and coop-eration already in place, the identification of victims and diag-nosis of their disease would almost certainly have been delayed considerably, and the consequences of that delay could have been severe.

Later work was to confirm cases of the same disease back to 1978, with convincing clinical evidence of cases back as far as 1959, none of which had been noticed as a new disease. It seemed like "just another cause of ARDS," to quote one clini-cian in the area. Isolated cases were easy to miss, and they had been overlooked.

The outbreak that killed Merrill Bahe and Florena Woody was different. Merrill Bahe's extreme fitness stood out as unusual. So did similar disease in four young people over such a short time. So did the fact that it killed two of the four, but it could still have been dismissed as "an unidentified illness."

What prevented that oversight? An alert clinician realized there was something different about these cases and brought them to the attention of the state authorities. The organiza-tional structure of the IHS and the fraternal cooperation of its clinicians facilitated a search for similar cases. Without these factors, we might still not know about hantaviruses causing dis-ease in America.

IHS epidemiologist Jim Cheek had initially been alerted to 5 possible cases of the mystery illness. By May 20, less than a week later, there were 10. On May 24, an alert was sent out to every doctor in New Mexico giving details of the new disease.

By May 26, 19 possible cases had been identified. Merrill Bahe was the youngest, the oldest a woman of 58. Twelve were dead. Not all were Navajo; in fact, one fatal case was in a woman from Iceland. However, all were from on or around the reservation.

On May 27, the *Albuquerque Journal* ran a story under the headline "Mystery Flu Kills 6 in Tribal Area." The press scram-ble had begun.

REACTION

The **Arizona Republic:** *"Navajo Sickness Probe Sought"*
USA *Today:* "NAVAJO FLU CLAIMS 11"

Across the country, newspapers, television, and radio were carrying stories of "Navajo Flu," the deadly new disease.

A group of Navajo schoolchildren excited about visiting their penpals at a private school in California found the invitation suddenly withdrawn. What now looks like racism seemed then, in the absence of any facts at all about the causes and effects of the mystery illness, like simple common sense. At that point, the high-profile victims were Navajo and no one knew how the disease might be caught.

From the proximity of those first reported cases, many people, including professional epidemiologists, assumed that the illness was spread from person to person and that the safest course of action would be to avoid people, principally the Navajo. That instinct was consistent with memories of other recent "plagues," including polio in the early 1950s and Legionnaire's disease in 1977, when health officials recommended avoiding public places. Through all this, there was precious little information on which to base decisions

Anglos weren't the only ones avoiding association with the Navajo. A family of Hopi dancers from Arizona, scheduled to appear at Mesa Verde National Park in Colorado, canceled their trip because they didn't want to cross the Navajo Reservation. The Hopi Reservation is completely surrounded by Navajo land; there was no other way out. They were trapped there for the foreseeable future, undoubtedly imagining the disease closing in.

A member of the Ute Mountain Ute Tribe was admitted to a Colorado hospital with a suspected case of the disease, and the local press jumped on that bit of information because it would have meant expanding the apparent boundaries of the outbreak. When that case turned out to be something else, the

Ute Tribe issued an unequivocal statement that there had been no Ute victims of the "Navajo disease."

Television programs such as "Good Morning America" and "Larry King Live" warned travelers to avoid the Four Corners because of the still-unidentified disease. Downtown merchants watched in amazement as a tour bus full of senior citizens drove down a Four Corners main street, all of its passengers wearing surgical masks. Tourism officials and tourism-oriented businesses began receiving inquiries about whether it was safe to visit the area. In an industry where failure to make hay while the summer sun shines results in a long, hard winter, locals obviously did not want to discourage visitation. While everyone tried to allay the panic, in private there was some recognition that it might not be a good time to invite visitors into the area. Rumors of a deadly disease were bad for business; the reality of an epidemic that struck down tourists as well as residents would have been far worse. The truth was that no one knew what to expect, what to do.

With school recessing for the summer, parents considered sending their children to stay with relatives outside what they believed to be the affected region. Others, not wanting to expose their children to anyone who might be infected and lacking any idea who that might be, kept them home and set them to performing useful tasks, such as cleaning out garages and basements. Later, they were horrified to realize what a mistake that could have been.

The problem was that no one knew what was causing the disease, and there were many possibilities. Some were more plausible than others; few could be ruled out without investigation. In the absence of concrete information, rumors were rampant.

SUSPICIONS

One of those rumors was that "the government" knew more than they were telling. In the western United States, the government is often seen as a specter, with an all-pervasive, mostly negative, influence. It is also a major employer in western states rich in public land, but in times of tension, some people tend to forget that the government is actually a neighbor who works for the Forest Service, a friend at the post office, the Bureau of Reclamation dam builder who sits in the next pew on Sundays. Instead, they think of nameless, blank-faced "men in black" sent from Washington on some secret mission that puts western-ers at risk.

That perception is not without foundation.

A long-standing rumor in the rural West has been that AIDS was a creation of the government, either an experiment gone awry or an intentional "plague" engineered to eliminate undesirable elements of society. Although the technology to engineer such a deadly virus does not exist even now, some credence was lent to the general idea when it was revealed that researchers had intentionally withheld treatment from 399 African-American men with syphilis for 38 years, up until 1970. Samples had been taken from them at intervals in order to study the course of that disease. It hasn't been that long ago since such "scientific innovation" was inflicted on the victims of World War II by both the Japanese and the Germans; only the naïve believe it could *never* happen here.

Native Americans had their own legitimate, although dis-tant, memories of such a travesty. In June 1763, Fort Pitt on the Ohio River was under siege by the Shawnee, Delaware, and Mingo tribes. To compound the troubles of the commander, Colonel Henry Bouquet, there was an outbreak of smallpox in the fort. The cases were isolated as much as possible in a "hos-pital" under the drawbridge. Colonel Bouquet, however, obvi-ously concluded that desperate times called for desperate measures.

In July, in a letter to Lord Jeffrey Amherst, the British mil-itary commander in North America, Bouquet suggested that he would to "try to inocculate the Indians by means of Blanketts that may fall in their hands" [sic]. During negotiations, the commander of the local militia, William Trent, "gave them two Blankets and an Handkerchief out of the Small Pox Hospital," hoping that they would "have the desired effect."

The attempt to "inocculate" succeeded, and the resulting epidemic spread across the continent, killing many thousands of Native Americans from at least six tribes, as well as substantial numbers of colonists. A biological weapon is always a two-edged sword.

The use of that particular weapon set a precedent for suspicion among Native Americans that would surface more than two centuries later, when a hantavirus emerged on the reservation where the federal government had forced the Navajo to settle.

That wasn't the only suspicion; at least two others weren't groundless either. In both, the culprit was the United States government.

War has always been big business in the United States, and during World War II, the atom bomb was big business in New Mexico. Although the project that developed the bomb was dubbed "the Manhattan Project," a great deal of it was carried out not in New York but in northern New Mexico, in a tiny enclave called Los Alamos on the Pajarito Plateau. The first bombs were tested on the White Sands Missile Range in southern New Mexico. Eventually the weapons tests were moved to the open, "uninhabited" deserts of Nevada and Utah—upwind from the Four Corners—and the radioactive fallout frequently drifted across the entire region. In the early days of those aboveground tests, residents were alerted not for safety reasons but so that they could go outside and view the spectacle for themselves. Mushroom clouds are an indelible memory for many children of the West. Herds of livestock suffered severe consequences of the radiation exposure; human beings did too, and some survivors continue to suffer, experiencing higher rates of cancer and other radiation-induced conditions. The legacy of radiation is long lasting and may not end with this generation.

Once genes are changed they are changed forever; any genetic mutations caused by radiation exposure cannot be undone and may be handed down.

Fission is the splitting of atoms, and the destructive power of nuclear weapons depends on having a very dense mass of atoms to split, releasing the energy contained in those atoms. A great deal of ore is required to produce a small amount of fuel for such a reaction, and a great deal of human energy goes into the mining, transporting, and refining of that ore. Some parts of the Four Corners region are rich in uranium, and during the Cold War, uranium mining was an important industry in those places.

The United States government possessed a considerable amount of information about the risks of such professions; in the interests of maintaining a state of national readiness, officials chose not to share that information with miners, millworkers, and truckers who were exposed daily to radon—the invisible, odorless, tasteless, chemically inert, but highly radioactive gas that is a product of the natural decay of uranium. When radioactive decay products are inhaled, they become trapped in the lungs. As they break down further, they release small bursts of energy that can damage lung tissue, leading to cancer and other respiratory illnesses.

Late in the 20th century, Congress issued a formal apology to the victims and passed the Radiation Exposure Compensation Act, to—as the name implies—compensate those who were unknowingly exposed to that radiation. More recently, there have been ongoing efforts to "lower the bar" and award money to people with a wide range of radiation-induced medical conditions. Many, though, were already dead.

Many of the uranium mines were on the Navajo reservation, and compared to other available jobs, work in the narrow, unventilated mine tunnels paid very well. As a result, many of those victims were Navajo.

So the Native Americans of the Four Corners had good reason to believe the United States government hadn't always had their best interests at heart. While few really thought the new disease was aimed at exterminating them, it was not outside the realm of belief that some previously benign microbe had mutated following exposure to radiation.

Radiation wasn't the only possible link. The U.S. government had recently agreed to destroy its store of chemical weapons, and some residents pointed—again upwind—to incinerators in Utah. Others pointed to the southeast, to Fort Wingate, New Mexico. Fort Wingate is a U.S. Army munitions depot. "Or at least that's what they *say* it is," conspiracy theorists muttered darkly. Researchers looked into that link and discovered that the wind had been blowing in the wrong direction. Long-time residents could have told them that it nearly always does.

Naturally, far-fetched theories abounded as well. The new disease was reputed to have originated from the alien spacecraft said to have crashed near Roswell, New Mexico, in 1947 or from a similar crash reported near Aztec, New Mexico, in 1948. This concept isn't too far from the medieval belief that influenza was caused by the influence of comets, an idea carried into the present day by the theories of the British astronomer Fred Hoyle. A connection between Anglo-touted childhood immunizations and the new illness was suggested. One member of another tribe suggested that the outbreak was a curse brought down upon the Navajo because of their disregard for the environment as demonstrated by the smoky power plants.

Many bizarre-sounding ideas contain a kernel of truth, however, and one of those discussed in coffee shops around the Four Corners was that the climate of the region had changed, which wasn't a new idea. Hard winters always bring with them stories from old timers about how every winter used to be that way. Everyone has an opinion about the existence and effects of global warming, and changes in features such as vegetation are wrought more often by human habitation than by climate change. However, the armchair theorists pointed out, there *were* those big lakes that didn't used to be there. Ideas were flying, fast and frequently furiously. Before the scientists could determine what caused the disease, however, they needed to know what it was.

CALLING FOR HELP

Although there was an obvious fear that the new disease was spreading, there was still no idea what the cause actually was. At the state level, none of the tests had shown anything. It was time to call for outside help. After a number of informal contacts, on May 27, the Centers for Disease Control (CDC) in Atlanta, Georgia, were formally asked to assist with the investigation.

The CDC is a unique organization, bringing together experts in all areas of human disease, and with a special interest in catching new infections and mysterious diseases. As a federal organization, however, the CDC cannot intervene in state matters unless they are invited. They were now invited.

To an outsider, the CDC is a daunting organization. With a multibillion dollar budget, laboratories handling the deadliest pathogens in the world on a routine basis, and a list of staff that reads like a "Who's Who of Infectious Disease," they seem able to do anything. These resources, however, have to be used to watch for any disease, anywhere in the world. There were at least 14 major problems occupying their attention in early 1993, from Milwaukee to Bangladesh. Added to this, at that time, the CDC was going through serious budget cuts, shedding staff, and was nearly paralyzed by a federal hiring freeze.

Responding to this outbreak was to require serious "horse trading" within the CDC to free up the personnel and funding required. In his book, "Virus Hunter," C. J. Peters, the head of the CDC Special Pathogens Branch, says "CDC was not going to let people die just because the budget was tight . . . We are essentially given a credit card with no spending limit when there's an emergency facing the American public."

The expertise that the CDC could bring to the scene was to prove crucial in identifying the mystery killer.

THE PRIMING OF ATLANTA

A meeting was called at the CDC for Friday, May 28, just before the Memorial Day weekend that closes down half the country. The meeting was chaired by emerging diseases specialist Dr. Ruth Berkelman and, even for the CDC, was big. Members of all eight divisions were present, covering everything from virus diseases to safety at work. It was to be a very wide-ranging meeting. Members of every division seemed to have the considered opinion that the cause was likely to be within somebody elses's area of expertise. Toxins, bacteria, viruses: all were considered. However, agreement was hammered out on how to handle the CDC's role, and responsibilities were assigned.

The field investigation was to be led by Dr. Rob Brieman, a bacteriologist and specialist in respiratory disease. Back in Atlanta, Peters was to run the laboratory investigations. A small team of epidemiologists was sent to Albuquerque immediately, under the leadership of Dr. Jay Butler. Samples began to flow back to Atlanta for testing.

ON THE GROUND

Jurisdiction between agencies is always a potential cause of conflict or at least confusion, and in the case of this outbreak, the agencies involved were numerous enough that problems were unavoidable. The Four Corners region includes, logically, four states, each with its own state health department. Add to that the jurisdictions of autonomous Indian tribes that contract with the Indian Health Service, a federal agency. Then add the University of New Mexico, the Centers for Disease Control, and a media frenzy that was threatening to get out of hand.

On top of all of that, there are very different attitudes in the different agencies. The CDC scientists came in to the area with little direct local knowledge and a strong sense that the outbreak had to be put into a national context. To those on the ground, this could grate, with the CDC team looking like they were more interested in epidemiology and abstract understanding than in the fact that people were dying. Some local providers, who had personal relationships with the victims, felt that CDC officials more than a thousand miles away were insulated from the pain and fear of local families affected by the disease.

It did not help when local health care workers and biologists were portrayed by the national media as hick yokels being rescued by the white knights from Atlanta, as in the case of the experienced field ecologist pictured in one newspaper as an "old Navajo trapper." However, everyone involved was aware of the real villain. They just did not know what it was.

ORGANIZING THE HUNT

The investigation of an outbreak does not just need scientists and clinicians. The CDC also sent press officers and fixer uppers with wide experience of field investigations. They needed offices, laboratory space, equipment to protect the investigators, trucks, and everything required to take samples and get them to Atlanta for investigation. Local teams needed to be trained in what was required. The delicacies of the situation needed careful handling. Despite the tensions inherent in such an urgent project, everyone went in with the best of intentions. No one wanted to harm the local cultures and economies, but clashes were inevitable.

LIFE GOES ON

While the investigators mobilized to deal with the new disease, local health-care providers were having problems of their own. Without knowing what the threat was, they had no way of knowing how to handle it. The only safe assumption was that the strictest of isolation procedures must be observed, which is difficult to accomplish in crowded hospitals with limited space and equipment. No one knew how fast the disease might spread or what treatments might eventually prove successful. Should they stock up on blood? On antibiotics? Antivirals? Body bags?

Meanwhile, they also had to deal with an influx of patients who did not have the new disease but who thought they might. Indicators were extremely broad—fever, aches and pains, flu-like symptoms—but providers didn't want to miss someone who might be exhibiting its earliest signs, particularly if it was highly contagious. They also didn't want to inadvertently expose people suffering from nothing more than fright to the disease. Hospitals exist to cure disease, but at some times, in some places, they can be epicenters for disease, bringing together the victims with those as yet uninfected and allowing a disease to spread within a community.

At some facilities, precautions went so far as to advise prospective patients to stay in their vehicles—usually cars and pickup trucks but also including horse-drawn wagons and school buses—and to have the clinicians perform a sort of triage there.

Privately, again and again, local physicians reviewed what they knew: local residents were contracting a disease they could neither identify nor treat, and a high percentage of those cases were fatal. People don't become doctors without learning some historical epidemiology, and so, in their darkest moments, some of them couldn't help envisioning what *might* happen. They could easily imagine quarantine notices on doors; the worst-case scenario involved military-enforced quarantines of thousands of square miles of the United States of America, and the political implications of that, particularly if those lines were drawn along racial boundaries, were mind-boggling. This disease seemed to be striking society's healthiest members; no one wanted to think about an epidemic so severe that it left no one strong enough to bury the dead. That possibility, while extremely farfetched, was not nearly as impossible as most modern Americans like to believe. It had been only 75 years since the Spanish flu killed so many residents of some mountain mining towns in southwestern Colorado that there were barely enough survivors to dig the graves.

Publicly, providers did their best to calm everyone's fears. There was, after all, no scientific evidence that pointed to imminent disaster. Of course, there was also no scientific evidence to prove that one wasn't on its way. As yet, there just wasn't much evidence at all.

3

UNRAVELING THE MYSTERY

· ·

Where observation is concerned, chance favors only the prepared mind.

LOUIS PASTEUR, ADDRESS GIVEN ON THE INAUGURATION
OF THE FACULTY OF SCIENCE, *University of Lille,* 1854

· ·

CONTAINMENT

Specimens from the outbreak started reaching Atlanta on May 31, including samples from the environment, from domestic animals, from rodents found near the dwellings, and of course from the victims themselves. They were not as thorough or as well organized as the researchers at the CDC would have liked: "poorly labeled samples in plastic jars," to quote C. J. Peters. They reflected the difficulties of working on the ground in the middle of an outbreak of lethal disease, but they were real, they were all that was available, and they would have to do.

There was an immediate problem with handling the samples. Infectious agents, be they viruses, bacteria, or anything else, are classified at one of four "containment levels."

Level One is "good laboratory practice": basic safety such as gloves and white coats, no more, used for agents that cannot infect humans or cause any other major problems.

Level Two is for known diseases of humans that are not a serious threat: common cold viruses, for example. Work is performed in a cabinet that deflects an airflow away from the user to prevent infection.

Level Three is for threatening, lethal diseases; the human immunodeficiency (AIDS) virus is one example. Samples are closed off from the user so that there is no contact.

Then there is Level Four. In Level Four, the most deadly agents are handled under extreme conditions. This is the level used for Ebola. Each worker in the containment laboratory works in a "space suit," with triple gloves and a filtered air supply. At the time of the outbreak in the Four Corners, there were only two fully equipped Level Four facilities in the country: at the CDC in Atlanta and at the United States Army Medical Research Institute of Infectious Diseases (USAMRIID) at Fort Detrick, Maryland. It is debatable whether there were any others anywhere else in the world.

The immediate question was how to handle the specimens from the Four Corners. Any one of them could contain unknown amounts of an agent that killed within days. Level Four would be safest, but it would mean that there were very limited facilities to handle the tests and very few workers trained to do so. In the words of C. J. Peters, "there is no way instantly to buy trained, experienced people," and both time and experience were essential.

It was decided to use Level Three containment for the work, with Level Four used for certain specific tests where the agent might be present at very high levels, such as trying to grow any virus present in laboratory animals. However, even Level Three requires strict containment and highly trained workers.

Because specimens in the field contain the same agent, the already fearful inhabitants of the area were treated to the sight of CDC investigators taking samples of their everyday environment while wearing what looked very much like space suits. Although there were extremely sound reasons for that practice—among them the protection of those inhabitants themselves—it wasn't very good public relations. It did look to some observers though the investigators cared considerably more for their own welfare than for those around them. The fact that those investigators worked for the federal government was not necessarily reassuring.

That didn't mean that the CDC workers had all the advantages. They were out in the desert summer sun wearing airtight masks, oversuits, gloves, and boots, but because they were deliberately looking in those places that might be hiding the agent that had already killed over a dozen people, the precautions were those that were required, by law and by prudence.

MEANWHILE, BACK AT THE LABORATORY

It was a busy time at the CDC. The horse trading had freed up some people to help, but for the key investigators, going home was to become a real luxury. Scientists with international reputations took to working the loading dock to get the specimens as soon as they arrived. People were dying, and the scientists knew that somewhere in those samples were the clues they needed to identify the killer. It was a time at once exciting, frightening, stimulating, and exhausting and the real reason why many of them were in science in the first place.

As the specimens came in, they were tested for any agent that could be the cause of the outbreak. Extracts of tissue samples were sent to the various laboratories for testing. Direct tests were used to find the genetic material of possible agents. To detect bacteria, they were spread out on a wide range of different nutrient gels. For viruses, they were inoculated into laboratory rodents, the best way to detect an unknown virus.

At the same time, blood from patients was being tested for antibodies using a range of stored material from possible infectious agents. If the patients had been infected, the antibodies in their blood would bind and could be detected—in essence, the footprints of a killer.

The first stage was to test likely candidates, agents known to cause pneumonia. Many of these had already been tested in New Mexico, but in order to be certain some were tested again, and the range of tests expanded. The second stage was to test agents that sometimes could cause those symptoms. The third was to test the long shots: everything else in the freezers.

The CDC investigators did have some hunches. The sudden onset and massive reaction looked like a chemical toxin, but the inflammation of the lungs was like that seen in some bacterial diseases where a specific protein, known as a superantigen, causes massive immune responses. Other indicators pointed at viruses, possibly an Arenavirus, a relative of the African killer, Lassa fever.

One pointer was an elevated number of white blood cells in patient blood samples. To C. J. Peters, with his extensive experience with viruses from all over the world, this looked like the effect seen with hantaviruses. Hantaviruses were only known to cause disease outbreaks thousands of miles away, on a different continent, and when they did, they attacked the kidneys. However, there was some hantavirus material in the freezer, so that was tested too.

All of the assays for any agent, likely or unlikely, were negative—until June 3, when the first assay for antibodies to hantaviruses was read. There it was: a weak but definite reaction, not huge, but enough to suggest that something related to the known hantaviruses had infected those patients. The next day another test system was used.

Four days after the first specimens arrived in Atlanta, the killer was identified: a hantavirus.

DISSENTING OPINIONS

Hantaan, the first hantavirus, was isolated from the Asian striped field mouse, *Apodemus agrarius,* from which it spreads to humans. Although the disease, a hemorrhagic fever with accompanying kidney damage, had been known for a thousand years, it was not until 1978 that the virus causing it was identified. The story of Hantaan and the disease, hemorrhagic fever with renal syndrome (HFRS), is detailed in Chapter 7.

Since then, other hantaviruses had been found. Only one seemed to cause disease outside Europe or Asia: Seoul virus, carried worldwide by the brown rat (*Rattus norvegicus*). If they caused any disease at all, it was the same kind as the first virus, Hantaan, but usually milder. Often they caused no apparent disease. The worst hantavirus outbreaks might kill one in five—bad, but nothing like the one-in-two mortality rate of the current outbreak.

The only hantavirus known that was native to the Americas was apparently harmless to humans and was carried by the meadow vole, *Microtus pennsylvanicus.* There were no meadows near the site of the New Mexico cases.

However, if the results were correct, there was a hantavirus attacking the lungs and killing over half of those infected. Unsurprisingly, not everyone believed the result.

It is not uncommon to find evidence of multiple infections in a sick patient. They can be either agents that have taken advantage of the weakened body or a nonspecific reaction with an enraged immune system throwing out anything it can in an effort to save itself. Many scientists thought that was what the tests were showing: an insignificant agent, secondary to the killer. Others suspected a totally irrelevant reaction, a "false positive."

However, there was a clue, and it was the best clue yet.

Elsewhere in the CDC were some of the ultraspecific reagents known as monoclonal antibodies. Unlike normal antibodies from blood, these are carefully created highly purified antibodies that detect only one specific tiny stretch of protein. These particular monoclonal antibodies had been created to detect one tiny bit of hantavirus. They were used on the samples. They found a hantavirus. And where they found it was in the tissues of the lung, where it would have to be to cause the disease that was killing people in the Four Corners.

WHAT NEXT?

The results said that the agent was a hantavirus, but the reaction of patient antibodies with known hantaviruses was weak. The outbreak was in the wrong place, with the wrong symptoms. Even though the monoclonal antibodies were picking it up, if it was a hantavirus, it looked like a new one.

Lurking in the recesses of the international databases of genetic information was the sequence of letters that are the shorthand for the genetic code of the known hantaviruses, and it was knowing these sequences that was to allow the code to be broken.

POLYMERASE CHAIN REACTION

In 1983 a new technique had been developed: the polymerase chain reaction (PCR). It was a technique that was to utterly revolutionize the face of biology.

The genetic code, the code of life, is written in just four letters: A, C, G, and T. These are the shorthand for the bases, the component units of deoxyribonucleic acid (DNA), the stuff of genes. In all cells, two strands of DNA carry the information that is used to make everything in the cell. The base on one strand dictates the base on the other by a code of opposites, outlined in Chapter 9.

A shorter-lived related molecule, ribonucleic acid (RNA), carries the instructions to the machinery that does the work, the structures and enzymes (catalyzing proteins driving chemical reactions) of the cell. Viruses are not cells, however, and while some carry their code as DNA, most use RNA.

In cells, genes are made of two strands of DNA. One strand is a mirror image of the other. Using two short stretches of synthetic nucleic acid "primers" and a heat-resistant copying enzyme, repeated cycles of heating and cooling split the two strands and allow copies to be made. By choosing two locations for the primers a short distance apart on the genes, the first heating and cooling cycle makes a copy. The second cycle copies the copy as well as the original. The third copies the copy of the copy, the copy and the original. The fourth . . . and so it continues, for 20 or more cycles per run. Because each time all of the copies are used to make yet more copies, there is a massive amplification of the short stretch of nucleic acid between the primers. After one run, the PCR will produce millions, billions, or even trillions of copies of that one part of the gene.

Because the primers bind using the code of opposites described in Chapter 9, they will only bind to the right sequence of bases. By altering the temperature and other conditions, they can be made less choosy, so that they will bind to something that is close to but not an exact match.

Hantaviruses are among the majority of viruses that use RNA, and with RNA a special enzyme is used to copy it to DNA, ready for PCR. Once the genes of the virus are copied, as long as the sequence is known or even half known, it is possible to look for them, copy them, and examine them in minute detail.

AMPLIFYING THE AGENT

Nine months before the Four Corners outbreak, the CDC had recruited an expert on the use of PCR, Dr. Stuart Nichol. It was to him that they turned next, and his expertise was to prove central to identifying the killer. Using the genetic sequences of known hantaviruses, Dr. Nichol designed primers to detect "conserved" parts of the gene sequence of hantaviruses of the two main classes. Because conserved regions do not vary much between related viruses, this method stood the best chance of detecting a related virus.

The two types of hantavirus known at that time were those that infect "Old World" rats and mice (*Murinae*) and those that infect voles (*Arvicolinae*). Hantaviruses from both classes were known to be in the United States. One was the first native American hantavirus. The other was the Seoul hantavirus, carried by the brown rat and found on every continent except Antarctica. However, they were both on the northeastern seaboard, thousands of miles away.

After some initial misleading results, a modified form of the PCR test came up convincingly positive. The next step involved some more horse trading. Dr. Nichol "borrowed" a machine that could actually read the genetic sequence of the amplified nucleic acid, sending one of his staff over to that laboratory at night when there was no one around. Reading the actual genetic code of the virus, they confirmed that they had a new hantavirus.

WHERE DO YOU COME FROM?

With the identification of the virus responsible, a lot of information slotted into place. By June 3, there were more than 20 suspected cases, but it appeared that one of the most terrifying possibilities probably was not going to happen.

Hantaviruses, as a rule, are not spread directly between humans. They infect each one directly from the source, and the source is rodents. More specifically, the source is the urine, droppings, saliva, and nesting materials of rodents.

Despite the worry over the possible spread of cases among the Woody family, there was now another explanation. Merrill Bahe and Florena Woody lived in a trailer that two different teams of epidemiologists had examined. Both had noted signs of rodents, many rodents. After the death of Merrill Bahe, Franklin and Jackie Woody had lived in that same trailer and had been exposed, in the same way, to the same infection.

In retrospect, it had been somewhat irrational of the populace to assume human contagion. Many of the Four Corners' most feared diseases are animal and/or insect-related: plague, vesicular stomatitis, rabies, and tick-borne diseases. Humans, though, tend to think of themselves as the center of the universe.

COYOTES, CARNIVORES, AND MEN IN SPACE SUITS

As soon as the initial identification was made, the next step out in the field was obvious. Hantaviruses live in rodents. Suddenly the rodents of the Four Corners had a new predator: men in containment suits. Instead of teeth or beaks they used small aluminum boxes containing all kinds of delicious rodent edibles. However, there was a small drawback to deciding to dine in these tempting new locations: the diner wound up over a thousand miles away in Atlanta, frozen solid. (Not always, though; coyotes found the idea of canned food very tempting and sometimes even managed to tear open one of the traps.)

Within a few months the CDC had 20,000 samples of animal or human tissue from the Four Corners.

GOING PUBLIC

On June 11, 1993, the CDC publication *Morbidity and Mortality Weekly Report,* commonly known as MMWR, carried the first fully informed report on the nature of the killer loose in the Four Corners. It reported cases covering all of the Four Corners states: 17 in New Mexico, 5 in Arizona, 1 in Colorado, and 1 in Utah. Not all of these held up through later laboratory testing. Of the 24 victims, 14 were of Native American origin. Twelve had died.

MMWR reported that the earliest case was from the end of 1992, with one confirmed case in March 1993, four in April, and nine in May, although those figures were revised later. The curve was still rising. That was a major cause of worry.

Although MMWR stated that "No restriction of travel to areas affected by this outbreak is considered necessary," this publication has fewer readers than the others that were reporting a deadly disease rampaging through the Four Corners.

By June 25, 12 of the cases reported earlier had been shown not to be due to hantavirus infection. Of the 12 that were confirmed as hantavirus disease, however, 8 (75%) had died, making the outbreak appear more lethal than ever.

REACTION

A 42-year-old rural Colorado woman with symptoms of the disease was admitted to a hospital emergency room on July 3 and died only 8 hours later, as physicians were attempting to stabilize her condition so that she could be transported to a regional medical center in Albuquerque.

By then, sudden death with flooded lungs was becoming almost familiar. CDC officials were speaking publicly about the suspected cause of the disease, dubbed (at least in the press, although it seems unlikely a journalist would have coined the phrase without hearing it from a medical source) "hantavirus-associated adult respiratory distress syndrome." They had released the information suggesting that it was spread by contact with rodent feces and/or urine and suggested that the Colorado woman might have contracted it while cleaning out a shed. The fear increased because mice are a common sight in the Four Corners.

North of the reservation boundaries, other details about this case caused increasing concern. This victim was a middle-class white woman, which was disturbing news to people who had convinced themselves they were safe because the disease struck only "poor" Native Americans. Furthermore, she had not been in New Mexico, and she had probably contracted the disease not in the desert but in a mountain valley.

Many residents of the Four Corners had managed, until then, to observe the outbreak with some degree of detachment. It had suddenly become much more real in the minds of those whose community was now a pin on a CDC map. The boundaries had been expanded to include residents who had thought it could never happen to them. As new cases were identified, that process would repeat itself throughout the region.

Suddenly, though, the media became a useful ally as well as a fear-mongering foe. The press began to do what it does best: disseminate the information that was finally available.

Public health workers issued advisories that began by warning, "Avoid all mice! Keep rodents, especially mice, out of the house." Residents were warned to seal paths by which rodents could enter dwellings, openings down to a quarter of an inch across, and to carefully avoid leaving out food, pet food, garden seeds, or anything else that might attract them. They were instructed to trap (but not poison) and dispose of rodents very carefully while wearing rubber gloves and surgical masks. Poisoning was not recommended because of the risk of mice dying in inaccessible places and continuing to spread disease. Mice dribble urine everywhere they go, but Four Corners residents well acquainted with rodents noted somewhat sarcastically that a spring-loaded trap snapping either on or near a mouse is likely to effect a more dramatic release of both feces and urine. Rodent excreta was to be cleaned up by soaking it in a chlorine bleach solution and then sealing it in double plastic bags. Breathing dust from mouse-infested places was to be avoided at all costs.

Most of these recommendations remain in force today, although recommendations about trapping rodents have been revised somewhat. Current prevention guidelines are printed in full in Appendix A.

After those stringent and alarming guidelines, residents were further instructed not to be overly alarmed. "If someone even just finds a mouse, they're really freaking out," the director of one county health department told a reporter, "and I just hate to see that happening, because the threat isn't that great. I just hate for them to get real upset any time they find a mouse because they're going to have mice around."

For precisely that reason, because mice are extremely common in the high desert region of the Four Corners, getting upset was just about all most people could do; there were only a few concrete actions anyone could recommend they take to reduce their risks of contracting the disease. Years later, that dearth of precautions remains. "Avoid rodents and their droppings" is the key to the possible safeguards.

PUBLIC EDUCATION

Health agencies also issued descriptions of "common symptoms" of the new disease, and those lists often included every symptom any ill patient might think to report. A health department news release from early July recommended that patients contact their physicians or hospital emergency departments immediately if they suffered from fever above 100.5°F, persistent cough, muscle aches, headaches, conjunctivitis, abdominal pain, vomiting, or diarrhea. Hotlines were set up, and daily updates were provided through diverse media sources.

Interestingly, many of the early advisories neglected to mention "difficulty in breathing" as a potential symptom of the disease, even though that was Merrill Bahe's primary complaint and was certainly a defining characteristic of the later stages of the disease. That oversight was soon corrected.

Many concerned individuals went one step further and researched the disease themselves, and what they found in the literature was a paragraph of long words that frightened them even more: myalgia, dyspnea, interstitial infiltrate, thrombocytopenia, hemodynamic instability, neutrophilia, atypical lymphocytes, and elevated serum LDH. Those terms either described the same symptoms health workers had listed or explained what caused them, but they were sufficiently disturbing to create a great deal of unease in a large number of people.

DEVELOPMENT OF AN EPIDEMIC

Such public information provided a large pool of "possible" cases that health-care providers had to sort through, and may have helped identify some cases. Statistics rose and fell as potential cases were identified and then confirmed or discarded (or, in some cases, confirmed, reevaluated, and then discarded). Although the publicity had in some ways added to the hysteria, some medical workers privately conceded that it had only touched on the realities of the nightmare. The medical community was no longer panicked, but its members were weary and depressed.

The pattern of illness had begun to diverge. One Four Corners state health department press release warned that "anyone who has had the initial symptoms for more than 4–5 days with no accompanying shortness of breath does not fit the classic definition of the disease; however, some of the suspected victims, including the most recent . . . have not conformed to this pattern." While 3 to 5 days is most common, we now know that it can take up to 10 days for this stage to develop. In some cases where symptoms did not fit, suspected hantavirus infection was later diagnosed as something else.

The same release stated that symptoms "quickly progress to acute respiratory distress," which, one physician cursed privately, "means they drown in their own fluids before we can do anything for them." That was the way it seemed to those trying to deal with it.

It was not a comfortable way to die. The victims succumbed either to the flooding of the lungs (pulmonary edema) or to heart failure caused by lung damage, stress, and hypoxia, the inability of the flooded lungs to provide sufficient oxygen. Nor was it comfortable for the health-care workers who could do little but stand by and watch it happen.

PUTTING THE
PUZZLE TOGETHER

· ·

*Memory performs the impossible for man; holds together past
and present, gives continuity and dignity to human life.*
MARK VAN DOREN, *Liberal Education,* 1943

· ·

It was now early July, and the worst fears had been allayed. Researchers had identified the agent of disease, they had some basic understanding of how it was transmitted to humans, and they were beginning, they thought, to learn how best to treat it, but there were still holes in the puzzle. They had pieces, sometimes more pieces than they knew what to do with; the problem was ordering them into a picture that made sense. Again, the questions were asked: Why here? Why now?

Why?

WHO KNOWS?

In some respects, the emergence of such a disease in the Four Corners (instead of anywhere else in the United States) could be considered a stroke of fortune. Because of the sparse population, relatively few people were at risk. The total population of the Four Corners states is barely more than 10 million; less than that of the metro Los Angeles area. Because of the network of communication between providers, the outbreak was identified relatively quickly. And because of the long collective memory of the area's traditional inhabitants, suggestions about the causes and controls of the illness were available, although their value was not recognized immediately.

Although the investigation of a new disease does involve white-coated scientists using state-of-the-art technology, most of the time and much of the resources are spent at the site of the outbreak, asking questions, taking samples, and examining the area where the infections are occurring. In this case, there were obvious questions to be asked.

EMERGENCE

The Navajo Nation is a vast and complex place. It is, in many ways, a Fourth World country, still developing, yet surrounded on all sides by the world's last remaining superpower. The United States itself is broad and varied. Anyone who has boarded a plane in Los Angeles or New York and stepped out onto a runway in the Four Corners has some sense of the scope of those variations. In this land of contrasts, newcomers are at a decided disadvantage in understanding the forces that hold life here in balance.

It is irresponsible to lump all Native American religions into one doctrine, but a theme that runs throughout many of them is the concept of "emergence," of progressing spiritually from one world into the next. The local inhabitants believed they had emerged into the deserts of the southwest.

Therefore, the topic of "emerging diseases" was politically difficult to introduce. This was not the time for science and religion to clash. No one wanted to draw parallels between traditional beliefs and the appearance of a deadly disease. No outsider wanted to suggest inadvertently that hantavirus was divine retribution on the part of *any* deity. In order to understand the outbreak, however, it was important to understand the events that had led up to it.

Mythology is the body of knowledge members of a culture pass down from one generation to the next to explain their understanding of the realities of their lives. Some social scientists hoped that by working backward through Native American's oral tradition they might find some clues about the outbreak. The Navajo had lived in the area for hundreds of years and as yet accounted for most of the cases. However, they have a traditional reluctance to talk of the recently dead, and they had been deeply offended by much of the media coverage, which seemed to blame *them* for the problem they were suffering. They believed that to speak of something bad was to risk bringing it down on their own heads. They were also private individuals, understandably suspicious of outsiders, particularly white government outsiders, and sensibly reluctant to have their lives examined closely by strangers.

The CDC investigators needed information only the local residents possessed, and they needed it quickly, but they had no status to demand it. The Navajo Nation is a sovereign entity, and the delicate political negotiations extended all the way to the president of that nation and a cabinet member of another. Donna Shalala, Secretary of the U.S. Department of Health and Human Services, issued a statement that the "sensitivities" of the Navajo would be respected. Navajo President Peterson Zah publicly urged tribal members to cooperate with the investigators. Privately, restrictions were undoubtedly placed on the outsiders. It was an awkward situation, and it seemed to some that the government was invading the reservations where, not too many generations before, it had interned the Navajo and their neighbors.

Local officials, including the employees of the Indian Health Service, had their doubts that a great deal of information would be quickly forthcoming. They knew from experience that relationships of trust develop slowly. The phrase "Indian standard time" is common in towns on and near the reservations of the southwest. Sometimes it is used in a pejorative sense; often it is an honest recognition that traditional peoples perceive time differently than those who participate in the commerce-regulated schedules of the modern world. There is a belief in the Southwest that everything happens when it is supposed to. Communication would be no exception.

A DRIP, A TRICKLE

The Navajo certainly did not want to associate themselves with the disease; in fact, they wanted very badly to disclaim any connection. Not entirely certain of the behaviors that might later be discovered to have put them at risk, they were not too sure of what they might be confessing to if they admitted that they or someone they knew had suffered from it.

Interviews were conducted with tribal elders, with medicine men, and and with anyone who seemed as though he or she might be able to offer information about any aspect of the outbreak. Interviewers went out to the pueblos to speak with people whose ancestors had inhabited the Four Corners long before the Navajo arrived.

Much of the information made more sense in retrospect. The more the researchers knew about the disease, the more information they could extrapolate from the interviews. Once they knew that rodents carried the disease, for example, they could ask relevant questions and fit that piece into the puzzle.

They could elicit information about food supplies, population changes from year to year, and connections to weather patterns. Looking back, the clues jump out. Most of the interviewers say it wasn't quite so easy at the time.

The process of synthesis undoubtedly worked in the opposite direction as well. As more details became available, more reliable information filtered out to the public. Individuals learned what symptoms were associated with the disease as cases were confirmed, and they were able to assimilate that with their own memories and oral traditions more effectively.

As in any mystery, some of the clues were undoubtedly false and many were somewhat suspect. The seeds planted by the investigators sometimes took weeks or even months to bear fruit; everyone hoped the results could be attributed to awakened memories and careful consideration. Sometimes, though, respondents cooperatively said just what they thought the researchers wanted them to say. Sometimes, no matter what they might be thinking, they said nothing at all. Among the researchers, the suspicion occasionally surfaced that some fun was being had at their expense or that the realities were shifting in a manner no outsider could ever hope to comprehend. The trick was to decipher their meanings and decide how much credence they deserved.

Dr. Charles Calisher, a hantavirus expert from Colorado State University working in the area at the time, speaks of searching for mouse kachinas among neighboring tribes. Kachinas are a part of the Puebloan Indian culture, masked representations of powerful forces that the traditional inhabitants peoples of the southwest see acting on their world. On his first swing through the region, he was greeted with blank stares. By subsequent trips, however, such kachinas were available.

What did that mean? Possibly it meant that researchers weren't asking the right questions. Possibly it meant that the residents of the region were taking their time in deciding whether and how to answer. Possibly it meant that they were mulling over the events of the recent past and developing their own interpretation, independent of the official researchers. Possibly it even meant that some were attempting to squeeze a few drops of profitable juice from the bitter fruit of blame.

However, those are all dangerous judgments to make for someone focusing on a few narrowly defined aspects of a population. Culture is a fluid substance; its value exists primarily in its ability to evolve. If the past were truly dead and had no relevance to the events of today, it would not be a part of that culture. The ability to retranslate history in light of new developments is essential to survival, and those translations are not always a language understood by outsiders.

Local clinicians fared somewhat better, though. They had the advantage of being familiar to their patients and could elicit information within the boundaries of an already established relationship rather than just appearing at someone's door asking questions. Slowly, it began to seem as though there was some memory of cyclical clusters of a disease very similar to the one that had been so unfamiliar to medical personnel when it emerged in this area in the spring of 1993. The pieces began to come together.

One Hopi individual told a journalist that he had heard stories of a "drowning sickness" that struck in years of plenty. When later asked to expand upon that story, though, he refused to discuss it, expressing a desire to disassociate his people from the new disease and its socioeconomic aftermath, and a reluctance to speak of the tales of his ancestors, fearing they would be misinterpreted by outsiders unaware, and uncaring, of their context. Other Hopis said the disease was unfamiliar to them.

As well as it could be patched together, some of the lore seemed to hint that the disease was seen in years when there had been a good harvest of nuts from the piñon pines, a favorite food of many of the wild rodents of the area and a nonperishable food that would last through the winter.

Obviously, though, the clues would not lead directly to a hantavirus. In his book, C. J. Peters says that Navajo wisdom identified 2 other years that had massive piñon harvests and huge numbers of mice: 1918 and 1933–1934. Some of those tales speak of sickness. Sixty to 75 years after the fact, it is difficult to evaluate that information, particularly because 1918 was the year of the Spanish influenza epidemic. The symptoms of the two diseases are in some ways very similar.

French-Canadian researchers noted a reluctance among the Navajo to associate too closely with *na-atoosi*—mice—and particularly to avoid sharing dwellings. They hypothesized a connection with hantaviruses. However, that connection may be tenuous. Rodents carry other diseases as well, most notably plague, and they also can deplete and contaminate human food supplies very rapidly. Even without hantaviruses, they would not be popular household companions.

The results of the interviews, while frustrating, were also informative in what they did *not* reveal. It had become apparent that there were no indelible memories of decimating outbreaks, which led to two possible conclusions. It could mean that the disease was not particularly virulent under most conditions.

Or it could mean that it really was new.

LOOKING BACK

Marietta Wetherill, the wife of an Indian trader who devoted much of his life to exploring the abandoned cliff dwellings and pueblos of the Four Corners, lived in southern Colorado and northern New Mexico a century ago. In the book "Marietta Wetherill: Life with the Navajos in Chaco Canyon," by historian Kathryn Gabriel, Wetherill related that the Navajo believed it was "the greatest of bad luck" to kill a snake, which is a sacred enemy.

Such prohibitions had bases in very sound logic. Snakes, especially the venomous rattlesnakes, are indeed powerful enemies.

They're also an integral part of the desert ecosystem. Like other predators, they are useful allies in any war against small rodents.

The concept of disease carried in the air was also known. Wetherill told Gabriel that the Navajo didn't like to live in Chaco Canyon, the crumbling ruins of a large ancestral Puebloan cultural center in northwestern New Mexico: "They said that the evil spirits make you sick, that the air was bad around the ruins."

PRIME SUSPECT

As early as late June, results from the testing of rodents were beginning to point to a likely source for the new virus. On June 25, MMWR published preliminary results of the rodent surveys.

The data were not surprising. "The Encyclopaedia of Mammals" states: "The North American wood mice of the genus *Peromyscus* have counterparts in the Murinae genus *Apodemus,* the wood mice of the Old World." The carrier for Hantaan virus is the Asian striped field mouse, *Apodemus agrarius.*

Results reported in MMWR showed antibodies to a hantavirus in rodents collected around houses in the outbreak area. If antibody was present, it showed that the rodent had had a hantavirus infection. A total of 191 animals of 12 species were captured. Thirty-four of the rodents tested showed antibodies to a hantavirus; 33 were *Peromyscus* mice.

Of 11 pinon mice (*Peromyscus truei*), 1 had antibody to a hantavirus. The rest of the catch was *Peromyscus maniculatus:* the deer mouse. Of 107 captured, 32 had antibody to a hantavirus.

The prime suspect had been identified.

ISOLATING THE VARIABLES

In a region where human population density is sometimes still measured in square miles per man instead of the reverse, rodents are much better adapted to the vagaries of desert life. Mice breed quickly and are highly mobile; as carriers of disease, they have quite a lot to recommend them. The deer mouse has an additional quality that made it a likely culprit in the emergence of a hantavirus: it is not shy. Unlike most other *Peromyscus,* deer mice show no reluctance whatsoever to enter human dwellings; they are quite comfortable sharing living space and food supplies.

Mice are always there. So what made this year different?

EL NIÑO?

The name El Niño (literally, a boy child, but a colloquial term for the Christ child) originated on the Peruvian coast. It was used to refer to a warm current that appeared around Christmastime. The name is now used to describe a huge movement of warm water toward the South American coast that has a far-reaching influence on global weather. In essence, it is a disruption of normal seasonal weather patterns, amplifying some and suppressing others.

Although the catch phrase "El Niño" has become an explanation for every variation in weather on the planet, it is actually a long-established weather system that has been occurring as far back as records exist. The name is appropriate in that cyclical climactic factors can bring either salvation or disaster to a subsistence economy; it is ironic, though, because the El Niño phase of the cycle is a negative force along the western coast of South America.

In order to understand what El Niño is, it is necessary to understand the factors that contribute to this great global cycle.

TRADE WINDS

Although winds are not as significant to mankind as they were in the days when all movement across large bodies of water was propelled by sail, the name of the trade winds is a reminder of those days. The oceans of the equator receive the most heat from the sun. As a result, the air above them is warmed and rises. Air flows in from cooler latitudes to replace the rising air. Because of the rotation of the Earth, the incoming air does not flow directly north or south but strongly westward as well as toward the equator, leading to the band of steady westerly winds driven by the turning of the Earth itself. In the Pacific, these steady winds lift an ocean.

A LUMP IN THE OCEAN

Because of the trade winds, the sea level of the western Pacific is actually about 1 to 2 feet higher than in the eastern Pacific. Not only is it higher, the trade winds also blow the warmer surface waters before them. The "normal" situation then is that in the eastern part of the Pacific, deeper water (which is colder than the sun-warmed surface water) is pulled from below to replace the water pushed westward. Along the South American coast there is an upwelling of cool water flowing from the Antarctic. This flow, known as the Humboldt current, or the Peru current, brings nutrient-rich Antarctic water to the fishing grounds off the coast of Peru and Chile, making them among the richest in the world.

However, this huge imbalance is not stable.

EL NIÑO

At the start of an El Niño event, the higher, warmer waters around Indonesia begin to flow eastward. Nobody knows for sure what the triggering event is. A failure of the trade winds, allowing the lump in the ocean to even out, is a likely cause, but why do they fail? Other factors that may be involved are massive movements in the deep ocean waters or storms from the Indian

Ocean pushing against the trade winds. No single factor is likely to be the sole cause.

As the warm water that had been propelled to the west by the tradewinds flows back eastward toward the coast of South America, it pushes down on the Humboldt current and the flow of nutrients is stopped. The Peruvian fisheries fail and huge numbers of seabirds die. At the height of an El Niño event, the warm waters are pressed against the shores of tropical South America, while unusually cold waters flow around the archipelagoes of the western Pacific.

The effect builds upon itself. Warmer water near the coast weakens the trade winds, which fail then to do their part to cool the ocean, which is further warmed and so further weakens the winds. This feedback cycle is what makes El Niño grow, in some cases, into a large phenomenon.

Water temperature has effects that reach far beyond the surface of the sea.

WATER AND WEATHER

The total temperature variation involved in an El Niño is only about 8°F, but the energy required to warm half of the surface waters of the equatorial Pacific ocean by even 1° is more than would be generated by the entire nuclear arsenal of the world. That much energy can have huge effects.

It is the energy contained in warm seawater that powers the great weather systems. Moisture evaporating from warm water is what provides the monsoon rains, so when the sea surface is cooler than usual, droughts follow. When it is warmer, violent and wet weather conditions result.

While the rich seas become a desert, the Peruvian desert blooms, with heavy rainfall and the germinating of seeds that have been waiting years for just this event. However, the heavy rain and strong winds also bring death in floods, in landslides, and from diseases such as cholera, dysentery, and diarrhea as rising waters contaminate drinking water and push people into crowded evacuation areas.

To the west, lands used to monsoon rains see drought and fire. The huge Indonesian forest fires of 1997 and 1998 were the result of El Niño. Australia also suffers droughts.

It is not just the lands at the ends of the current that are affected. The eastward movement of the warmest weather results in large changes in the global atmospheric circulation, which in turn can bring changes in weather to regions far removed from the tropical Pacific. The jet streams in the upper atmosphere, so important to weather in the temperate regions of the world, are directly affected. Although the broad reach of the Indian Ocean lies between Africa and the Pacific, the 1997–1998 El Niño brought extensive flooding to eastern Africa, with rainfall reported as being up to 20 times normal in some areas. The rains were followed by huge numbers of mosquitoes breeding in the floodwaters and a lethal epidemic of the mosquito-borne Rift Valley fever.

In the United States, El Niño means different things in different places: flooding on the California coast and greening of the high deserts of the interior Southwest, with droughts in the Pacific Northwest. The effect is very variable and is never certain, even in one place. Meteorology is a science of estimates and probabilities, not certainties.

EL NIÑO/SOUTHERN OSCILLATION

All things come to an end, and El Niño events are no exception to the rule. The return of cold waters to the South American coast is part of the same cycle. Produced, essentially, by the reversal of the factors that created the El Niño, this event is known as La Niña (the girl child). Strong La Niña years often, but not always, occur after El Niño years.

The whole cycle of warm and cold water flows is known as the El Niño/southern oscillation (ENSO) and lasts from 3 to 7 years. Most El Niños are short, lasting a year or two, but some-times they can last longer or run in a series with only weak La Niñas or even none at all in between. According to the United States National Oceanic and Atmospheric Administration, it is unusual for El Niños to occur in rapid succession, but that was the case during 1990–1994. That cycle was linked to the han-tavirus outbreak in the Four Corners.

The power of different El Niños and La Niñas varies. Some are weak, with limited effects, whereas others produce far greater change. One of the most powerful El Niños known ran from 1997 through the spring of 1998.

ENSO cycles are part of the normal cycle of the planet, and considerable effort goes into prediction and monitoring. A string of temperature-monitoring buoys floats across the width of the Pacific, and the curious can see the results in real time on the Internet. However, even the experts cannot say what any one event will mean at the local level.

OFF THE MAPS

It hasn't been too long since the settlement of North America huddled against her coasts and the interior was called, only half-jokingly, the great American desert. The implication was that it was a cultural wasteland, with few people and fewer ideas gathered there. That was never true and it's not true now, but certain realities remain. The Four Corners seems extremely sparsely populated to someone who lives in New York or Los Angeles, or perhaps even Atlanta. Because the provision of goods and services is most profitable when targeted on population centers, this area receives little attention. Weather forecasting is a standing joke among inhabitants; weather maps skip over this region as if it didn't get any weather at all. Weather does happen here, however, and it varies considerably.

Deserts are so named because they are dry, not because they are empty. That dryness may be the only factor desert ecosystems have in common. Every year, tourists come from great distances to stand on the peaks of the western mountains. From there, they can look out across vast expanses of a landscape that falls away in every direction. Distances are deceptive for those who forget how many dimensions are there. Fewer than 30 miles west of the 13,000-foot peaks of the La Plata Mountains in southwest Colorado, one has already dropped more than half of the vertical distance to the Pacific Ocean, which is still three states away. From the tundra above the tree line, descending through the tall pines, the aspens, the scrub forests of piñon, juniper, and oak, into the grasslands, and then into the bare rock and sand that the word "desert" evokes for most people, the precipitation figures don't change all that much.

Deserts focus life near sources of water. That doesn't always mean *running* water; the attraction may just be a marshy bottomland, a green highlight in a landscape dominated by shades of brown. That focusing effect is temporal as well as spatial because desert life exists largely in potential. Life in the desert is a hugely complex cycle of resources jealously hoarded and judiciously used. Within hours of a nourishing rain, the desert can spring to life, demonstrating complexities unimaginable to those who've only seen its latent phases. Gloriously green plants appear, seemingly from nowhere, and across the entire spectrum of desert life every living thing goes about collecting and storing the resources essential to its survival. The growing season is short; this year's rain often contributes to next year's crops.

That dramatic change can be brought into full flower by very small amounts of moisture. The average annual precipitation in northwestern New Mexico, for example, ranges from 5 to 10 inches. In the mountain communities, it rarely reaches 20 inches per year. The high mountains receive more but certainly not much, especially compared to the coastal rain forests of the Pacific Northwest.

So, in the desert, the difference between a drought and a flood is measured, literally, by the inch. That difference can also be in the timing.

Deserts aren't always hot places; winters in the southwestern desert are both cold and windy. Moisture that falls as snow may be biologically useful. If it falls on frozen ground and is sublimated—drawn by the dry winds into the atmosphere without ever even becoming liquid—it will not provide much benefit to the biological community. If, however, the sun shines the next day and warms the reddish, sandy soil so that the snow melt soaks in, that same snow has a different result. Even when the air temperate is well below freezing, the solar gain on dark soil, at altitudes of a mile or higher and under thin, clear air, can make that precipitation available . . . if, again, the sun and wind don't evaporate it.

The rest of the year, precipitation patterns are equally fickle. Torrential rains can turn into torrential floods, bypassing nearly completely the local community of flora and fauna. Rain in autumn has a different effect than rain in the spring. Rain at the proper time of year feeds neatly into the cycle of photosynthesis and food production that extends all the way up the food chain. Rain at the wrong time just runs downhill to the sea.

Although there are very apparent seasonal fluctuations in precipitation, the feast-or-famine cycle is not consistent throughout the region, which is—geographically as well as ecologically—a very broad place. The long El Niño cycle of the early 1990s has been well documented, but its predicted effects did not hold true throughout the Four Corners.

Throughout most of New Mexico, for example, 1992 was a wetter year, with more precipitation falling earlier in the summer, longer and higher monsoon peaks, and more moisture in the fall. Precipitation remained somewhat high going into the spring of 1993.

In Colorado, though, the variations were not so apparent. A significant drought had plagued the region beginning in the spring of 1989; water supplies did not even reach average levels until late in 1990. They fell again until the winter of 1991–1992. Conditions were wet in the first months of 1992, had some peaks in the spring and later summer, but were very dry again in autumn. The surface water supply index, which measures, essentially, the water available for agriculture, including that stored in reservoirs, did not rise substantially above normal until February of 1992, and it wasn't until March that the Colorado Division of Water Resources decreed that southwestern Colorado had an abundant supply of water. Utah showed a similar pattern. The effects of El Niño seemed nebulous.

Still, the Native American reservations are the places that would logically experience the greatest effects of fluctuating weather patterns. They received the least rainfall on average (which may have been, in part, why they were available to be made into reservations in the first place) and they had the least land under irrigation. Droughts would be felt most severely there; increased precipitation would bring the most dramatic positive changes to the most arid lands.

THE FORGOTTEN LANDS AND THE PROMISED LAND

A thousand years ago, the Four Corners was the province of the ancestral Puebloans who would inhabit the cliff houses and grand pueblos for the next few hundred years. They domesticated animals and grew crops on the mesa tops. Archaeologists have uncovered evidence that they built check dams and storage basins to capture water for agricultural and household use, but the extent to which they could control their environment was limited. By and large, and for very good reasons, they accepted the limitations the desert placed upon them.

Shortly before 1300 A.D., the ancestral Puebloans abandoned their canyon homes and moved southward. Various theories have been proposed to explain their abrupt exodus, and the most accepted is that a combination of factors convinced them it was time to move elsewhere. They had been suffering a long and severe drought, and it is likely the resulting famine was accompanied by disease. These factors may have been interpreted as a strong indication that their gods had other plans for them.

The tribes that moved into the area in their wake were hunters and gatherers, although they too eventually settled down to subsistence agriculture (the only kind there is, as any Four Corners farmer or rancher will confirm). They, too, accepted the realities of life in an arid land.

The conquistadores and the friars crossed this area, but didn't put down roots. From the south, the Spanish influence was increasingly felt, but the empty deserts were unsuitable for agriculture, and no mineral wealth presented itself for the taking. In the 1860s, though, U.S. Army troops led by Colonel Kit Carson destroyed the crops and flocks of the Navajo and then forced approximately 8000 of them on the "Long Walk," 300 miles to Fort Sumner, New Mexico. Thousands died during the march and their subsequent imprisonment; by 1868, the Navajo had agreed to accept reservation life. Carson and his contemporaries inflicted similar conditions on members of other tribes. The result was the opening of vast (and very harsh) sections of the West to white settlers.

Although the view of Native Americans as "noble savages" served no one very well, it was true that the new settlers were not as willing to believe that the land could not be tamed. Most of them came from Christian traditions and believed that God had given them dominion over all the earth. They apparently also believed that such control brought with it ownership as well as (or, all too often, instead of) stewardship, and they naively believed the desert could be forced to accommodate them.

The Mormon pioneers were sent out with carefully conceived plans to create settlements and bring land into production. That meant bringing water to crops; there was no other way. That was a good thing then, and it's not "bad" now; it did, however, change the ecology of the West. Where there is more food for humans, more humans will come. There will be more food for mice as well, and the mouse population is very much dependent on the food supply. A growth cycle had begun; a new balance would have to be achieved.

DREAMS COLLIDE

So what happened in 1993?

The weather had changed, and—in a very simplistic analysis—more moisture meant more food, which meant more mice, which meant more opportunity for disease to spread from mice to humans. While such weather events are cyclical within spans of no greater than a decade, something else had happened.

The West had changed; the population of the Navajo Nation and other rural areas was increasing, which moved people into places previously inhabited only by smaller animals. Those settlement patterns had changed humans' exposure to mice and therefore to hantavirus.

It was inevitable that those two worlds would come into increasing conflict. It happens not only with mice; rural residents and recreationists are experiencing more snakebites, more mountain lion attacks, and more bear scares. There is no longer anywhere for those species to retreat when they perceive themselves threatened by the advancement of human beings.

Perhaps, though, nature has her own ways of maintaining balance.

5

OF MICE AND MEN

· ·

*I'm truly sorry man's dominion, Has broken nature's social
union*   ROBERT BURNS,
          To a Mouse, On Turning Her up in Her Nest, 1785

· ·

"PARMENTER ESTIMATES THE MOUSE POPULATION, FEASTING
ON PIÑON NUTS AND GRASSHOPPERS, GREW 10-FOLD BETWEEN
MAY 1992 AND MAY 1993"   *Science,* 5th November 1993

"WHEN THE MYSTERIOUS EPIDEMIC BROKE OUT, THESE SCIEN-
TISTS KNEW THE DEER MICE HABITS AND HABITATS; THEY ALSO
KNEW THAT THEIR NUMBERS HAD MULTIPLIED 10-FOLD FROM THE
PREVIOUS YEAR"   *The FASEB Journal,* Vol. 9, October 1995

"THERE WERE TEN TIMES MORE MICE IN MAY 1993 THAN THERE
HAD BEEN IN MAY OF 1992"

                    Centers for Disease Control
                hantavirus information website, 1998

But

> "AS FOR THE "TENFOLD RISE" NUMBER, I SUSPECT THE SE-
> QUENTIAL GENERATIONS OF NEWS REPORTS DISTILLED THE AC-
> TUAL, ORIGINAL INFORMATION DOWN TO A MORE TIDY FIGURE
> THAT, THROUGH REPETITION ALONE, HAS BECOME THE NUM-
> BER OF CHOICE."   Dr. Robert Parmenter, 1998

Another of the known facts about the 1993 outbreak was the 10-fold rise in deer mice around the outbreak sites.

It didn't happen quite that way.

OF MICE AND PLANTS

There was an El Niño event feeding the warm, wet weather in the southwestern United States and there had been local wet weather, but what did that mean?

In most parts of the Southwest there was a big increase in the amount of vegetation through 1992 and 1993. A wet year was followed by a mild winter, and in the spring of 1993 the arid lands of New Mexico were green. Among the vegetation that was unusually lush that year were the piñon pines. An often-repeated idea is the "mouse–piñon nut connection": that many piñon nuts mean many mice.

The year 1992 had been a "mast year" for piñon trees. In such a year the harvest of nuts in the fall is many times heavier than normal, and in 1992 there were so many cones that nuts were still reportedly left in the spring of 1993. Mast years are not unusual, however, and can occur every 5 to 10 years. Although mice will happily eat piñon nuts, they will actually eat almost anything, from insects through fungi, through all kinds of seeds to, occasionally, each other. Mice, like other rodents or insects, are often the link between vegetable and animal kingdoms in the food chain.

Adaptability is one of the main features of a successful animal, which is one reason why there are more rats than pandas. So the piñon nut crop is more of a marker for a very fertile time rather than the single explanation for all that followed.

Still, the rains in 1992 produced a lot of vegetation. A mild winter, followed by a wet spring in 1993, ensured that plenty of food remained available. There was a lot of food for anything that ate it. And mice did.

MICE, MICE AND MORE MICE

In deer mice, pregnancy produces four or five pups on average and lasts 3 to 4 weeks. The babies are ready to breed at 5 weeks old. There are usually three breeding cycles a year, but a warm winter and early spring can add in an extra one, tripling the number of mice that can be produced in that year.

Humans and mice are obviously different. Humans produce few offspring and then take great care of them, making sure that each one has the best possible chance to grow through a long childhood to maturity.

Mice do it differently. They produce large numbers of offspring, of which only a few may make it through to breeding age, even though that is only a few weeks after their birth. Mice do not plan their families. Every pregnancy produces about four new mouths, whether there is food for them or not.

When there is no food, they die. It may seem cruel; more significantly, for a mouse struggling to feed itself in the desert, it may seem wasteful. However, mice exist in competition with every other animal that eats the same kind of food. Given that they eat almost anything, that is a lot of competition.

What this breeding pattern means is that when there is food available, the new mouths are already there, waiting, ready to take advantage of it before some other species can. Then they survive in greater numbers, and breed within a few weeks. Mouse numbers can go up very fast indeed when there is enough food to permit it.

MICE!

In the real world, it's called rumor. The scientific establishment calls it "anecdotal evidence," and there was anecdotal evidence of large numbers of mice in the Four Corners area. It doesn't matter how many mice you see, unless you're doing it scientifically, it's "anecdotal evidence."

Many people living in the area were reporting seeing mice in numbers and places that were far beyond the norm. Even the investigators at the site of the first "index" cases of the new hantavirus disease in New Mexico had been surprised by the amount of rodent activity there. However, it was not scientific data when the investigators were told this, or to know that it was likely given the rich food supplies. Hard numbers were needed.

That information was important not just for hantaviruses. Other rodent-borne diseases, including plague, are cyclical and are possibly linked to the El Niño cycle of mild, wet winters that aid rodent population growth.

SEVILLETA

About 60 miles south of Albuquerque, in central New Mexico, is a unique place.

In 1817, in the town of Belen on the Rio Grande, a magistrate of the Spanish colonial authorities granted the lands known as Sevilleta to a group of families. In 1848, most of what was to become the state of New Mexico came under American rule. In 1912, New Mexico became a state. Along with the rights and privileges came something new: property taxes.

The old families fell into default, and the Sevilleta lands passed to General Thomas B. Campbell from Montana, who acquired the land by paying the back taxes. Many years later, the Campbell Family Foundation and the Nature Conservancy passed ownership on to the United States Fish and Wildlife Service, with the requirement that the land be used as a reserve and for environmental studies. On January 1, 1974, the Sevilleta National Wildlife Refuge (NWR) was created, and the land was closed to livestock grazing.

The Sevilleta NWR covers approximately 220,000 acres, spanning the width of the Rio Grande valley and the mountain ranges to either side: the Los Pinos Mountains to the east and the Sierra Ladrones to the west. The Rio Grande, the railroad, and Interstate 25 run down the center, and the refuge spreads out to either side like the wings of a butterfly.

In the 1980s, long-term ecological research (LTER) programs were created in order to obtain basic information about the American environment. Situated at the junction of three different ecosystems, the Sevilleta NWR was an obvious choice for an LTER program because one site allows study of a wide range of ecologies. Running in from the northwest is a plateau supported by the Rio Colorado. This is not the same Colorado River that carved the Grand Canyon; *that* Colorado River lies on the other side of the Continental Divide from Sevilleta. In the south of the refuge is the Chihuahan desert, studded with creosote bush. To the east is the edge of the Great Plains shortgrass prairie. The land looks harsh, but it is rich with a huge variety of life.

The Sevilleta LTER program was established in the fall of 1988. In early 1993, scientists based at Sevilleta and at the administrative center in Albuquerque were continuing their studies of the ecology of the area. However, very suddenly, one small aspect of their work was to be in great demand.

THE 10-FOLD RISE

A "rodent bloom" is a sudden large increase in the number of rodents. Was there a rodent bloom in progress in the Four Corners?

There was a sudden and very urgent need to know about mouse numbers, not just because there was an outbreak under way but because there was something very worrying about what that outbreak was. What was known about hantaviruses was based on studies of hantaviruses in Europe and Asia—Hantaan and Seoul in Korea and China and Puumala in Scandinavia—and with all of these, most cases of the disease occurred later on in the year. Numbers in the Four Corners were still rising. There could be a major epidemic on the way.

Even if numbers started to go down again, it was known that with Hantaan there are two peaks of disease each year: a small one in spring and a much bigger one in the late fall. If that were to happen in the Four Corners, the worst, by far, was yet to come.

So there was a real need to know just what was happening, and close to the area where deaths were occurring, there was Sevilleta, studying, among other things, rodent numbers, using the same aluminum traps that were to see so much use by the CDC teams.

Within a few months after the outbreak began, the name of Sevilleta LTER program manager, Dr. Robert Parmenter, would be known across the country. Unfortunately, what he said would become a little more garbled. The information is detailed, but it bears repeating.

The Sevilleta scientists assembled their information and published it on July 13, 1993: Sevilleta LTER Publication No. 41. The report contained information on the numbers of different types of rodents, from mice to chipmunks, at six points, within four areas of the refuge, covering the three different ecosystems, as well as different elevations. It included sites from desert to woodland, and all of them had mice.

Also in the report was information collected at four sites in Canyonlands National Park near Moab in southeastern Utah. The information ran back several years, giving solid baseline information for any recent change.

However, for no rodent of any kind was there a 10-fold rise within the last year. In fact, on all of the Sevilleta sites, not one deer mouse was trapped in the first half of 1993. There was a general population increase in related mice, including the white-footed mouse *Peromyscus leucopus,* the cactus mouse *Peromyscus eremicus,* the piñon mouse *Peromyscus truei,* and the brush mouse *Peromyscus boylii.* Some of these types of mice would later be shown to be infected with the new hantavirus, but none of them were the deer mouse, *Peromyscus maniculatus,* the main suspect.

At one Sevilleta site, high up in the Los Pinos mountains, the numbers had risen to seven times those seen in 1992. But overall, the number of *Peromyscus* mice at Sevilleta rose to 2.5 times the numbers seen a year previously—hardly a 10-fold increase.

At the Canyonlands survey sites, deer mice were seen; they were quite common. However, Canyonlands data showed only a one-and-a-quarter times the 1992 numbers of deer mice overall, with three times the 1992 numbers at one site. At two sites, numbers had actually fallen. So had the total number of *Peromyscus* mice trapped, to four-fifths of the 1992 level.

The picture sketched by those 2 years' worth of numbers was not as complete as everyone assumed. Left out of the information reported in the popular press were data on whether the 1992 populations used for comparison came from a bloom year themselves (in which case a twofold rise would be extremely significant) or a trough year, in which there had been extremely low populations. Everyone except the scientists themselves assumed that 1992 had just been an "average" year; few members of the public realized that such populations are always in flux.

Actually, Sevilleta falls outside the region normally defined as the Four Corners, and Canyonlands was 200 miles from the focus of the outbreak, but the data were solid for the sites examined. Dr. Parmenter's team laid it all out in detail, and the scientists at the CDC and in New Mexico took it for what it was: an indicator, from an area close by. It was the best data they had, but it did not demonstrate a 10-fold increase of rodents at the site of the outbreak.

Again, in Dr. Parmenter's words: "As for the 'tenfold rise' number, I suspect the sequential generations of news reports distilled the actual, original information down to a more tidy figure that, through repetition alone, has become the number of choice."

That was a diplomatic way of describing the distortions that had been introduced at the hands of the press. Others suspect that somewhere in those "sequential generations," some journalist had seized upon the number 10 not because it was accurate but because it was dramatic and offered an "easy" answer to a complex question: Why were people dying?

The Four Corners region has very few large communities. The most sizable, Farmington, New Mexico, had a population of fewer than 35,000 in the 1990 census. Most had fewer than 3500 inhabitants; many had fewer than 35. It is tempting to assume that the news outlets—newspapers and radio and television stations—in the smaller communities perpetuated the inaccuracies. That theory makes sense for a number of reasons. Small papers and broadcast media have fewer resources to devote to news gathering and so would logically be more likely to use second-generation sources of information: other, larger publications. Local reporters were extremely unlikely to have contacts at the CDC, for example.

That doesn't seem to have been what happened, however. In fact, local news agencies seem to have been cautious, for several very good reasons. For one thing, they had learned to be somewhat circumspect in dealing with sensational-sounding aspects of the story that had created negative consequences for their communities. By the time the mouse data became widely available, the outbreak was over and many small-town reporters had moved on to other issues. Those who did report it mentioned "marked" or "dramatic" increases "reported" in rodent populations. Perhaps because they were actually in the Four Corners, they were in a better position to realize how many, many rodents a 10-fold increase would actually involve and to understand that the population boom would manifest itself in other ways as well. More attuned to the regional ecosystems (as well, perhaps, as to the concept of ecosystems in general), they were somewhat skeptical that only one portion of it would flex without the others. The oversimplified cause-and-effect chain reaction of rain–piñon–mouse–virus–death appeared less simple to those who understood the context in which it had to take place.

It wasn't small-town journalists on tight deadlines who created the myth; instead, it was the national media that took the number and ran with it. *Science* is a highly respected journal, with a high-powered scientific readership. In the November 5, 1993 edition, however, as well as saying: "the mouse population, feasting on piñon nuts and grasshoppers, grew 10-fold between May 1992 and May 1993," *Science* also stated that "at the Sevilleta Long Term Ecological Research site near Albuquerque . . . . deer mice . . . . were everywhere." They weren't. However, if a respected scientific journal said it, there was very little chance that mass-circulation media would do a better job of it.

The fact was, in Bob Parmenter's own words: "The extrapolation to the Four Corners area was simply the best estimate available based on our Sevilleta experiences. The only real question at the time was 'did the rodents increase in this area prior to the epidemic?' The probable answer was yes, *if* the resident populations behaved the same as on the Sevilleta. Spatial variability in mouse populations is very high, so without data it was at best a 'general' answer to the question."

Dr. Parmenter's team was close to the right place, at the right time, with solid scientific evidence that supported the suggestion of an increase in rodent numbers in the Four Corners. It was enough. For the time being, it had to be. An extended program of trapping was begun at a hugely expanded range of sites throughout the Four Corners, with sampling every month instead of twice a year. Now the information would be solid.

TRIAL AND CONVICTION

"Identification of *Peromyscus maniculatus* as the Primary Rodent Reservoir for a New Hantavirus in the Southwestern United States" is only part of the title of a scientific report on the work done by the CDC and local teams that long, hot summer of 1993. Scientists like long titles.

However, that paper really had something to say. The teams had trapped 1696 small mammals of 31 species at 12 sites in New Mexico, 4 in Arizona, and 3 in Colorado. Almost half were deer mice; there were many deer mice in the Four Corners. They also trapped other related mice, rats, chipmunks, prairie dogs, squirrels, eight unlucky rabbits, and one skunk. Skunks can fit through very small holes, but precisely how a skunk fits in a trap designed for mice was not made clear. The person who opened it probably did not feel like explaining.

The rodents trapped were tested for antibodies to three different hantaviruses: Puumala from Europe, Seoul (found worldwide, mainly in Asia), and Prospect Hill, the only American hantavirus. Unsurprisingly, by far the largest number had antibody to Prospect Hill. Ten types of rodent and one rabbit tested positive.

Over 30% of deer mice had antibody, showing that they had been infected by a hantavirus similar to Prospect Hill. As yet there were no specific tests for the new virus, but the evidence was clear: guilty. *Peromyscus maniculatus* had been tried and convicted.

Of the related mice, almost 20% of piñon mice (*P. truei*) and almost 6% of brush mice (*P. boylii*) had antibody. By numbers and by blood testing, however, it was the deer mouse.

One problem with naming the deer mouse as the villain was, in the words of Dr. Parmenter, "it's cute." Deer mice are 4 to 8 inches long, half of that tail, with big ears and big eyes, brown fur on top and white underneath. It's much easier to blame a rat.

Another problem is what it meant for the rest of the country. The range of the deer mouse is huge, encompassing almost all of the United States except for the deep South and the eastern seaboard and extending south in Mexico and northward into much of Canada. That was bad news. The range of the host species was not going to limit the range of the new disease very effectively.

As mentioned earlier, another characteristic that set deer mouse apart from other *Peromyscus* species was its lack of shyness. Other mice tend to avoid humans and their habitations, but hiding out in the brush is not for deer mice, not when there are houses and outbuildings full of potential meals. They do not mind at all sharing their living space with the owners of that food. That made the confirmation seem like even worse news.

But of course the deer mouse was not a villain. It lives quite comfortably with its hantavirus and suffers no ill effects. It is pure chance that this particular virus can hop to a nearby ape: *Homo sapiens sapiens*. Man. And in man, it kills.

HANTAVIRUS IN THE MOUSE

Human beings are of very limited importance in the life of hantaviruses. Even with Hantaan, the first hantavirus identified in humans, it is difficult to grow the virus from a human source, but from the rodent host the virus is recovered easily. With the

American hantaviruses, no recovery of live virus from a human has ever been documented, but again it can be grown from rodents.

What this means for the way the disease develops in humans is explained more fully in Chapter 13. However, it is very clear that these viruses circulate in the host rodent independently of human infection and that our contact with the rodent ecology is what exposes us to the virus. From our human-centered point of view, it is difficult to understand that diseases as devastating as those caused by the hantaviruses are, basically, side effects to life in a mouse, but they are.

Understanding the life of rodents provided the information needed to tie down the cause of the new disease. Although much is known about the rodents that host these viruses, we still don't understand all of the factors involved. The main thing we don't understand is how the virus, so devastating in humans, apparently doesn't harm the mouse at all.

With Hantaan, the virus is passed between mice by breathing infected material. Because the virus is mainly in the lungs of the mouse, this is not surprising, although the virus does also appear to be present in the saliva, urine, and feces. Once the mouse is infected, it takes 10 days for the infection to establish. Even when the virus is present at high levels, the mice do not develop any apparent sickness. Hantaan virus circulates in their blood for a short while, but the mice produce and release very high levels of virus for several months. Although the mouse produces antibody, a powerful reaction against the virus, it does not clear the infection. While the level of virus the mouse releases drops, infectious virus can be present in the urine, feces, and saliva of the mouse for the rest of its life. It is a hazard to human health for all of that time. The bigger and older the mouse, the more likely it is to have antibody to Hantaan.

The Asian striped field mouse *Apodemus agrarius* is the main host, but several other types of rodent have been found to have antibodies to hantaviruses, although they have not necessarily been linked to human infection. This is common with almost all hantaviruses. Although there is one major host, other rodents, and sometimes other animals entirely, can be infected. In this, mankind is just an alternative host.

In the case of Hantaan and Seoul hantaviruses in Asia, 67 different species have been found to have antibody, showing past infection. Almost all of them will be infected but not able to pass on the virus. A few closely related species may be able to, but probably at lower levels. There is also very limited evidence that Hantaan virus might be found in mites on the rodent host, but this does not seem to be a main route of infection. Unlike other members of the same virus family, the *Bunyaviridae,* which includes Rift Valley fever and many other threatening viruses, hantaviruses do not seem to be able to be spread by insects or mites. For humans, this is one of the few good things about them. It decreases their chance to infect us.

A LOT OF RODENTS MAKE A LOT OF VIRUS

The two peaks of infection per year seen with Hantaan are mirrored by the number of Asian striped field mice, and the main, fall peak occurs when mice exhaust their available supplies of seasonal fresh food and invade human houses and buildings, seeking stored food. The numbers of these mice have been boosted by intensive agriculture, increasing human exposure to them, and so increasing the risk of Hantaan infection. Similarly, hantaviruses in Sweden have been linked to the number of their host rodent.

In the case of the European Puumala hantavirus, where the normal host is a small vole, moose, bats, and birds seem to be infected as well as humans, but again they are unlikely to be able to pass the virus on.

Voles and their cousins, the lemmings, have regular "boom and bust" cycles, with huge variations in the number of animals. Lemmings do not actually fling themselves from cliffs in dramatic mass suicides as many people believe, but the huge numbers of lemmings that can result at the peak of the cycle do lead to large numbers of deaths. The same is true of voles, including the bank vole, *Clethrionomys glareolus,* the main host for Puumala virus; variations in the numbers of this vole are closely linked to Puumala disease in humans.

COMING TO AMERICA

Only very recently has information become available on what the American hantaviruses do to their host rodent. Studying mice in the wild is difficult, but it made several things clear. The percentage of mice with antibody is far higher in males and increases as they get older. How it is spread is not clear, but the best guess is that it is passed by large males, probably in the saliva by "fighting and biting." The mice do seem to live quite closely, sometimes even turning up in the same trap together. In winter they apparently share burrows, possibly for warmth, making transmission of the virus more likely.

What is clear is that the level of infection in mice is quite low when there are only a few mice around, sometimes dropping below detectable levels. However, there is a "threshold" population level above which the number of infected mice increases sharply, possibly because population stresses increase contact between mice, and crowding boosts the aggressive, violent behavior that spreads the virus among mice. It was this that triggered the high levels of infection in mice in 1993, in which about 30% of mice were infected; in some high-density settings, almost three-quarters of all mice can be infected. If there are only a few mice, the risk is low, but as the numbers of mice increase there is a sudden sharp rise in the risk of human infection.

It also looked like not all areas were the same. It was already known that sub-populations of deer mice living at different altitudes had differences, for example, in coat color. It was now to become clear that they also had different levels of infection with hantavirus. Mice in the very lowest lying land, mainly desert, had lower levels of infection, as did mice at altitudes above about 8000 feet. In between were the highest levels of infection. This is unlikely to be due to any single factor. Variations in the mice themselves, in living conditions, in the amount of time each year during which they can breed, and in the density of mice in local areas are all likely to be involved. Unfortunately for residents of the Four Corners, there are many houses and towns between 5000 and 8000 feet altitude, including the Littlewater home of Merrill Bahe and Florena Woody.

LIVING TOGETHER

One thing that did seem to be the same as with other hantaviruses was that the virus did not harm the mice. As with Hantaan, after infection, the virus is found at high levels for a few months, then drops away but probably does not drop to zero. If that is true, the mouse may be able to pass on the infection for the rest of its life. It is a potential killer until the day it dies, and maybe even for a while after that.

How the virus manages to remain infectious in the face of the mouse's immune system remains to be discovered, but it seems that the virus throttles back its own growth inside the mouse. How and why? Those answers are unknown as yet.

In addition to not harming the mouse, one study showed that infected brush mice (*Peromyscus boylii*) seem to live longer. This virus and the mice have had 20 million years to adapt to each other. They seem to have done it well.

STUDYING THE HOST

Working with mice in the wild is tricky. They can and do refuse to cooperate with the study, and in the wide open spaces of the

Southwest, they have plenty of other options. It is much easier if the researcher can control the living conditions of the mice, and the normal way to do this is to take them inside an "animal house," where the mice are kept in climate-controlled cages under carefully controlled conditions of diet and environment. However, early work at the CDC in the normal animal house was inconclusive.

Infected mice can amplify the amount of virus present hugely. For safety reasons, all the work with infected mice at the CDC was done at the very highest safety level: Biosafety Level Four. That required space suits, triple gloves, filtered air, the whole shooting match. While these precautions are very effective at keeping lethal viruses away from the investigator, they are very, very difficult to work under. It is hard to work with animals at the best of times. Under Category Four conditions, it can get close to impossible.

Added to that, the mice were a long way from the southwestern desert, and it showed in their behavior. They did not like the animal house, and they did not adapt well to life behind bars. The attempt to study deer mice inside, in Atlanta, was not a success.

So, on the northwestern fringe of the Sevilleta refuge, something new has taken shape. Variously called "The Hantavirus Study Site," "The World's First Outdoor Category Four Lab," or "The Very Large Mouse Array" (derived from the name of a nearby radio telescope), it is a unique facility.

The first stage uses steel fenced 20-meter-square enclosures, containing 34 ready-made burrows constructed out of state-of-the-art 5-gallon buckets. Unlike normal burrows, these can be opened up to let researchers into the nests. These enclosures are used to quarantine mice and for studies of transmission of the virus. The next stage of the work uses much larger plots, 200 m on a side, containing native vegetation and again studded with desirable mouse residences. The facility is of huge value in actually understanding how the virus actually lives in mice.

Even the first stages of the work produced valuable information. Captured mice to be introduced into the enclosures were put in quarantine to ascertain that they were not carrying a hantavirus, and one pregnant female developed antibody where she had had none before, showing that she had been infected very recently. The mouse was perfectly well, even though she had virus protein at very high levels in her internal organs, including the heart. There was no sign that the virus had passed to the baby mice.

Work at the Very Large Mouse Array will produce much more information in the near future on how the virus is actually maintained in the mouse population. Such studies take time, though, to produce verifiable results.

From what was known in 1993, there was good reason to believe that high mouse numbers meant human disease in the Four Corners. So what happened?

WHAT GOES UP MUST COME DOWN ... BUT WHEN?

Good weather increases the food supply, which in turn increases the rodent population, but that correlation has its limits. Other factors will reverse the trend, including predation, diseases amplified by overcrowding, and increased aggression. For example, predators tend to be bigger than what they eat. As a result, their numbers tend to increase more slowly. As mouse numbers rise, more survive predator attacks because there are not enough predators to go around. However, when the number of mice starts to drop, for any reason, predator numbers are still rising. There are many new, very hungry predators helping to push those numbers down even faster. There's a cycle; there's always a cycle, but when would it reach its peak?

LATER THAT SAME YEAR

Well-nourished mice, breeding in mild weather conditions, will produce many more mice. In optimal years, they may even add a breeding cycle. More mice meant more virus and more human contact, and no one knew what would happen that autumn.

If the new hantavirus was to follow the same pattern as the European or Asian hantaviruses, then the number of cases would increase in the fall as the numbers of its host increased and they came into closer contact with humans. Nobody knew by how much the number of human victims would increase, and when you are dealing with a disease that kills half the people it infects, that is something you do want to know.

In Asia and in Europe, the fall increase in disease is attributed to animals "hunkering down next to people" when it gets cold, and the Four Corners has cold winters. During those winters, people get colds and flu, and the new disease caused symptoms that mimicked those of familiar maladies.

In winter the number of people showing up with symptoms that were almost certainly something else, but could just be the first signs of the new disease, would become very high indeed. Normally, all they would need was simple medication and rest, but not if they had hantavirus. The last thing anyone wanted was to send someone with the new, deadly disease home with some Tylenol. So they needed to know if it was going to strike.

Once again, attention turned to Dr. Parmenter and the Sevilleta team. They took samples in October, just before any increase could be expected. This time the study looked at the Pecos National Monument near Santa Fe in northern New Mexico. Again, it was not a site in the Four Corners, but one close by where information on numbers earlier in the year was available. By now, the "villain" was clearly identified, and they were on the alert for deer mice.

Something else had changed. Instead of working with what they believed were harmless little rodents, they were now hunting a killer. Shirtsleeves were out. Space suits were in.

Now, unusually, there was good news. Mouse numbers were dropping, although not massively, in the "crash" that can follow a rodent bloom. There was no sign of the fall peak in mouse numbers seen for the Asian field mouse that hosts Hantaan, which is the peak that leads to the fall outbreak of disease.

Although limited to this one site, the report concluded: "Rodent populations in the region have undergone significant reduction since the spring of 1993 . . . . The risk of human–rodent contact has been substantially reduced."

Nobody relaxed, but at least the information they did have was not threatening. Still, no one knew for sure whether a fall peak of disease was seen with this virus. Sure, there may be less mice, but what if they all decided to come into the warm? There were still enough to infect many people.

6

AT LAST, A PLAN

································

I wanted to live . . . Of course I did. I didn't want to leave my family. They needed me. But I was just so tired . . . I was just so tired. HANTAVIRUS SURVIVOR

································

MINIMIZING EXPOSURE

Now that both the virus and the host had been identified, the inhabitants of the Four Corners had some idea of how to protect themselves from exposure. In some parts of the region, principally the Navajo Reservation, that is indeed what happened. A systematic program of education and risk reduction was undertaken by the Navajo Nation and the Indian Health Service. It wasn't enough to tell people they had to keep mice out of their dwellings, sanitarians had to teach them how best to do it, which was a difficult challenge in rural settings more hospitable to mice than to humans. Educational materials were prepared. Home visits were made to ensure that they were understood. Supplies to aid in controlling rodents were made available.

The objective was extremely basic: deny rodents access to the places where they could expose humans to hantaviruses. Some of the more traditional Navajo, however, were not convinced that the cause was quite so simple. Their view of the world was a more holistic one, and the mice had been there as long as humans could remember. It didn't make sense to blame them for a disease that wasn't as much a part of the landscape as the mice were.

The concept of rodents as hosts for serious diseases was not foreign to the inhabitants of the Four Corners, but the education effort was complicated by the fact that hantaviruses generally have no apparent affect on the mice that carried it. Plague causes periodic and very obvious die-offs in the prairie dog colonies from which it emanates; with hantaviruses, that confirmation was lacking.

Regardless of the evidence, it clearly was not going to be possible to control the virus by eliminating the host. If annihilating *P. maniculatus* had been possible, the plan would have had its advocates. That wasn't going to happen, though. The range of the deer mouse is enormous, covering a large part of the continent.

It wasn't even possible to reduce their numbers much. Throughout the entire West, there are hundreds and often thousands of mice per square mile, and many of them are *P. maniculatus.* They occupy their own niche in a complex community of plant and animal life, part of a food chain with plants and insects below them and snakes, raptors, and carnivorous mammals above. In this region so sparsely populated with humans, when human ingenuity was pitted against the rodents' instinct for survival, the rodents had all the advantages.

The best that could be hoped for was to hold the mice at bay. Just trapping those within buildings would not be enough; there was a seemingly infinite supply waiting to take their place. Those inside would have to be exterminated, whereas those outside would have to be kept out. That doesn't sound difficult, but humans have been trying to just do that for all of recorded history. Still, on the reservation, a great effort was made to eliminate food sources for mice and to seal all routes by which they might be entering dwellings. In addition, people were educated about what to do if they did find a mouse or a nest.

Off the reservation, the risk was taken somewhat less seriously. These people, too, had lived around mice all their lives and had never been harmed by a hantavirus infection; why should they worry now? Because researchers could offer only theories about why the outbreak had occurred, many Anglos remained unconvinced that they were at risk. The attitude of many was extremely cavalier because, in most people's opinion, hantavirus was much like lightning: "If it's gonna get you, it's gonna get you, and there's nothing you can do."

Indeed the level of risk did seem similar, but most Westerners do have sense enough not to go golfing or mountain climbing in a thunderstorm.

Public health officials attempted to instill a similar sense of caution in dealing with mice. After all, the risk of being struck by lightning can be close to 100% for someone standing in the wrong place at the wrong time; in most other circumstances, however, it's virtually nil. In most situations, the risk of contracting a hantavirus infection is extremely remote, and in the situations where risk did exist, it could be managed.

Part of the difficulty lay in the way medical care is provided in the United States. On the reservation, the Indian Health Service is the principal provider and is, both in the way it functions and in the way it is funded, a governmental agency. Essentially charged with the responsibility for providing all health services to the entire Navajo population, it already possessed the structure and the contacts to undertake a wide-ranging prevention campaign.

In the private sector, which operates on a fee-for-service basis, though, the picture was different. Individuals choose their own medical provider, who can then admit them to the local hospital. Until that need arises there is a limited relationship between provider and patient. Individual states maintain health departments, with care provided by units in individual counties, but those also had a restricted clientele. There was no single agency with an established conduit through which to feed information to all the residents of the Four Corners.

Slowly, though, behavior did change. It was very calming to learn that a few amazingly inexpensive precautions could effectively reduce the risk of exposure. Disinfectants, mouse traps, and steel wool to block holes were all readily available; no special technology was needed. An ounce of prevention is worth a pound of cure, and when there is no cure, prevention is priceless.

BLAMING THE MESSENGER

The media attempted to do their part, and large amounts of airtime and ink were devoted to informing the public about the risk, prevention, and symptoms of hantavirus. Although necessary, it was not a popular service. Tourism is a vital part of the economy of the Four Corners, and news of the outbreak had frightened away many visitors. Merchants dependent on that source of revenue turned their frustrations on the messengers, and the only journalists to whom they had easy access were those who worked locally.

That hostility, although understandable, was less than logical. Potential visitors reevaluating the advisability of traveling to the Four Corners were not likely to base their decisions on a small-town newspaper or radio station; they were getting their information from the national media: CNN, *USA Today,* or *The New York Times.* They (and their travel agents) were also calling chambers of commerce and health departments. Chamber spokespeople attempted to allay their fears, pointing out that while the deaths had been widely reported, there had actually been very few cases of the disease. Health officials had to be more circumspect; they were only beginning to understand the risks. A fall peak in cases was still considered a possibility.

There is no doubt that the economy of the Four Corners suffered, although sales tax and lodger's tax statistics do not bear out the tourism industry's perception that "the hantavirus scare brought the 1993 season to a screeching halt." That is what locals called it, a "scare." No one wanted to acknowledge out loud that the outbreak had been fact, not fiction.

In the early 1990s, southwestern art was very popular. Interior design reflected the colors of the desert: sand, sage, and turquoise sky. Navajo rugs and Mission furniture were in demand, as were less authentic items of décor such as howling coyote figurines and turquoise-inlaid cow skulls. *Ristras,* strings of dried chilis, were chic ornaments for doors and kitchen walls, along with garlic braids.

The "new" southwestern cuisine was taking its place beside the more familiar "Mexican" food, and gourmands everywhere were experimenting with beans, chilis, tortillas, and, ironically, piñon nuts. Western wear was fashionable, and Native American jewelry was an integral part of the look.

In addition, southwestern archaeology was receiving increasing attention as Americans disenchanted with the present looked toward the past for answers. New Age adherents were also focusing their attentions on "vortex" sites in the Four Corners.

Those trends were still in their ascendency in early 1993, and merchants who were expecting a banner year were in for a rude shock. One Farmington waitress spoke of being able to look from one end of the main street to the other without seeing a soul. Although that may be an exaggeration, it captures the hollow feeling of a boom gone bust many communities were experiencing at the time the outbreak's shock wave hit their tourist season.

Some places fared better than others, and the difference may have been the border of the Navajo reservation. The misperception was (and, to a great extent, still is) that this was an Indian disease. It is ironic that while such erroneous thinking did not save victims and indeed may have put some people at unnecessary risk, it may have slightly mitigated the effect on tourism-oriented businesses in towns farther from the reservation. Some visitors who did make the trip turned back at the reservation line and spent their money elsewhere.

Resentment toward the media remained for 5 years after 1993, when health officials were warning that another outbreak might be on its way. Owners said their tourism businesses still had not recovered from the last "scare." That analysis reflects some important facts of life in the travel industry.

Tourists are fickle, and tourism is cyclical. For a while, the desert is "in" and then suddenly demand shifts to the beach, the rain forest, or urban destinations. Human beings can act very much like herd animals; diverted from their goal of the Four Corners, many stampeded off in another direction. That, more than the one "bad" year, may be the true effect of the hantavirus outbreak on the Four Corners economy. The upward trend was slowed and momentum was lost. In some communities, the difference may simply have been between expectations and reality.

In Cortez, Colorado, for example, tax figures show slow but steady increases in summer revenues throughout the early 1990s, and 1993 is no exception. Even that year, even during those months, gross sales increased. That does not mean that individual businesses were not badly hurt. Communities with broad-based economies fared much better than those more dependent on tourism revenues. Those locales and those businesses where visitation had not been well developed as a source of income would suffer the least.

LEARNING TO TREAT THE DISEASE

By late summer, the mortality rate had dropped from an initial high of 80% to below 50%. Working in conjunction with the CDC, physicians had developed a protocol that included fluid management as well as ribavirin, an antiviral drug.

Even though the virus was known to be a hantavirus, this was a very different disease to the hemorrhagic kidney disease (HFRS) seen with hantavirus infection in Asia and, in a milder form, in Europe. Hemorrhages were not seen, and the virus attacked the lungs, not the kidneys. The lungs were given support to get oxygen into the blood and to stop the strain on the heart. Giving fluid to counter shock was traditional, but in the new disease, something else was needed: diuretics to keep fluid from building up in the body and pressurized oxygen to keep the lungs working and ease the choking fluid back into the blood.

RIBAVIRIN

Ribavirin (Virazole) is used against a wide range of viruses, but unlike most antiviral drugs, exactly how it works is not clear, even to specialists in the field. It has been used successfully against other "exotic infections," most notably hemorrhagic fevers, including Lassa fever in Africa. Growing the Asian hantavirus Hantaan in cells treated with ribavirin showed that it was sensitive to the drug. In mice, ribavirin blocked virus growth. In specially selected mice where Hantaan did cause some disease, ribavirin cut the death rate.

It was judged to be worth trying in humans, and in 1985, the Chinese did just that. The first trial was on 57 patients, already with the disease, treated for 1 week with ribavirin. A larger trial on 187 patients was carried out the next year. The death rate was cut from 7.8 to 2.3%. Kidney damage, the main marker of HFRS, was reduced, as were the skin hemorrhages known as *petechiae,* the markers of hemorrhagic fever. Some side effects were seen, mostly an anemia, but ribavirin was saving lives. The Chinese are now one of the world's main manufacturers of ribavirin.

Ribavirin had been approved in the United States for use in its aerosol form against respiratory syncytial virus, which causes a flu-like disease that generally strikes young children. In 1993, it was being tested for use against hantaviruses. With a hantavirus killing people in the Four Corners, the CDC arranged for it to be made available, to be given by drip into the bloodstream. It was stocked at the Northern Navajo Medical Center in Shiprock for distribution throughout the region.

Its use in the Four Corners outbreak was based on hope rather than on hard evidence. Patients were arriving for treatment in the later stages of the disease, when any benefit from the drug was very unlikely. But it was the best best chance there was: it was the only antiviral available that showed the potential to be effective against the outbreak. Later work was to show that the new hantavirus was sensitive to the drug when grown in flasks of isolated cells, but it didn't work in patients. There was a very slight improvement in survival, but it was well inside the limits of random chance. Ribavirin itself is not harmless: anemia and other side effects were seen.

In the words of the CDC, "We don't have any evidence that it changes the course of the disease." In the words of a clinician in the Four Corners who was dealing with dying patients in the 1993 outbreak, "Ribavirin was useless." Ribavirin has still not been shown to have any clear-cut benefit for HPS, although studies on giving it as early as possible are continuing. It is likely that improved survival resulted from improved understanding of the course of the disease and appropriate treatment of the symptoms rather than from ribavirin.

CRITICAL CARE

Even among clinicians there was conflict with the white knights from the CDC. The initial guidelines issued by the CDC were described as "less than helpful" by that same doctor, who also commented: "knowing that it was hantavirus . . . didn't really aid in the treatment plan. The ones who survived were those who got good basic medical care in the emergency room and intensive care unit." That basic medical care was mostly supportive care: preventing secondary infections and supporting the body's functions while the patient recovered.

There is no denying the critical role of the CDC in identifying the virus that caused the disease and how it was spread, but it's also true that there was an occasional taint of bitterness. Physicians who contacted the CDC for information about treating HPS were given information on the CDC's current recommendations, which were evolving as more information became available. The CDC was the command center, able to collect information from diverse sources and evaluate the efficacy of various treatments, then report back to the clinicians with the latest data. Once notified of those recommendations, physicians weren't eager to incur the liability associated with violating official CDC protocols.

However, the "experts" weren't always there when patients died, despite the recommended treatments; local doctors were left explaining to family members what had gone "wrong" and why it had happened so fast.

What most rural physicians attempted to do whenever possible was to stabilize suspected hantavirus patients and transport them, preferably to the University of New Mexico Medical Center in Albuquerque. The primary reason for that was because that UNM had the facilities and the expertise that smaller facilities could not offer. Private gallows humor, which was not always tactful during the stressful summer of 1993, suggested another reason: nobody wanted to be left holding the body bag.

THE FRONT LINES

The CDC might have had the experts, but physicians in the Four Corners had the patients. No matter how skilled and dedicated those doctors might be, they were not practicing medicine in metropolitan Atlanta but in small, isolated clinics and hospitals. Telephones and computers facilitated the nearly instantaneous transfer of information; the transfer of patients, however, was not so easy. In 1993, definitive diagnosis of a hantavirus infection took days or even weeks because samples had to be sent elsewhere for testing. That amount of time was a luxury hantavirus victims did not have, and their attending physicians had to make decisions about how and where to treat them.

The treatment itself was not a pleasant thing to witness. It is never easy to watch someone fight for every breath. Hantavirus victims were frequently in severe pain and had to be sedated for the respirator. Families members asked why patients could not be given higher doses of pain medications, but such drugs carry their own risks: depressing bodily functions and stressing the liver and kidneys.

Early in the outbreak, it had become apparent that the survival rate was better at large regional hospitals, particularly at the University of New Mexico, where both equipment and expertise were more readily available. A patient could not be transported if his condition was not stable, and hantavirus infection was an unstable condition. Air transport was not always readily available; helicopters and fixed-wing aircraft were stationed centrally and had to be dispatched to rural areas, adding to the delay. Those resources were not devoted solely to hantavirus disease, as always, there were other emergencies occurring at the same time.

Other issues were involved as well. Shipping a critically ill patient to Albuquerque was a tacit acknowledgement that his survival was in question. Family members could not travel as quickly, and some of them could not travel at all. Theoretical advantages in treatment had to be balanced against the psychological disadvantages of separating a possibly terminal patient from his loved ones: sending someone who was very likely to die to a place where he would die alone. No one had forgotten that Merrill Bahe had died on his way to the hospital; everyone knew it could happen that quickly. Those choices were not abstract; they had to be made by human health-care providers for human patients.

Local clinicians could not view their patients as statistics; they were individuals, and their symptoms had to be handled on a case-by-case basis. Successes were exhilarating; failures were personal. Hantavirus infection was not the only problem in physicians' case-loads; other medical problems continued apace.

They were too busy to talk, and had they not been, they were reluctant for other reasons. The fact that the identities of those struck by the new disease were known so quickly across the nation made health-care workers uncomfortable about the lack of confidentiality. Because of that personal focus, most declined to talk to the press about the larger picture.

THE VICTIMS

During the summer of 1993, firsthand accounts of hantavirus were difficult to obtain. For those victims who did survive, the recovery process was slow and there was a definite stigma involved. It became clear relatively quickly that the disease struck Native Americans and Anglos alike, or at least in proportions that could be logically attributed to their contact with the host rodents. Not only did it cross ethnic boundaries, it crossed income lines as well. No one, it seemed, was immune.

Regardless of all evidence to the contrary, though, it was to remain, in many people's minds, the "Navajo flu." It was associated, however inaccurately, with poverty and with substandard living conditions. It was not, and still is not, a disease most people want to admit they've had.

One victim tells the ironic story that she had sworn that if she recovered, she would work to correct those misconceptions. She tried, she says; she spoke to friends, neighbors, and her family. Nearly unanimously, they urged discretion; they, too, did not want to be associated with the disease. She quit speaking out and now does not allow her name to be used in conjunction with hantavirus.

The story she tells in rare private conversations is gripping. She began to feel feverish and achy and believed she had the flu. When the aches and pains grew more severe, she sought medical attention and was hospitalized before the respiratory symptoms appeared. She, too, speaks of drowning, of perceiving a great weight on her chest, and a great exhaustion. She speaks of wanting to see her children one last time, and then of her mixed emotions about being sedated.

"I wanted to live," she said. "Of course I did. I didn't want to leave my family. They needed me. But I was just so tired . . . I was just so tired."

She did survive, and sometimes, she says, she still grows so weary that she realizes she'll never fully recover from her encounter with the virus.

"I used to think doctors could fix anything," she says. "Now I know they can't, and I know they probably shouldn't try."

That doesn't mean she ever gave up, she said, but she admits she can understand how other victims might. "It's the most horrible feeling: the tubes, the liquid in your lungs, the choking. You don't want to die that way, but you know you can't live that way either."

Few other victims are willing to talk publicly about their experiences. They acknowledge that the prejudices are unfortunate, but they aren't sure they can change that state of affairs. They will, however, give bits of advice:

"Go to the doctor right away. It's better to be embarrassed than to die."

"Pay more attention to your surroundings. It's not enough to notice the mice; you have to notice where they've been."

And perhaps the most poignant: "Don't think it can't happen to you. That's what I thought."

THOSE LEFT BEHIND

Family members of those who died of hantavirus infection are reluctant to speak openly as well. Those with traditional beliefs don't want to risk the same fate by speaking of it. Those who don't fear that feel a sense of resignation.

"No matter what you say, people will believe it was her fault, and it can't happen to them. She didn't keep her house clean enough, they say. That's not true; you could feed your baby off the floor. It could happen to anybody."

That's a very accurate perception. People will believe the victim was at fault and that they are different because it gives them the illusion of safety. Middle-class people want to believe hantavirus is a disease of the poor; mice and viruses, however, are no great respecters of money. Town dwellers want to believe it's a rural disease; to a mouse, however, a wide green lawn is sufficient acreage. Educated people want to believe the greatest single risk factor is ignorance, and they are right, but degrees are no protection. Instead, what's needed is recognition of the true risks.

Those risks are very real, but they're not very great. They can be avoided, and sometimes nature helps out.

DECLINE AND FALL

There was real fear about what was going to happen in the fall of 1993. So what did happen?

From the start of the outbreak, there was a steady increase in the number of cases each month. On March, 2; April, 5; May, 6; June, 10; and July, 12. Of those 35 cases, 20 were fatal. Nobody knew whether the numbers would go on increasing. If they did . . . .

In August, however, there were only three cases and two in September. Then there was a nervous time as the numbers rose again in October. Six cases—was this the start of the much feared fall peak?

No. November and December had only one case each. There was no big fall peak in 1993, but of the 48 people who developed the new disease in 1993, 27 were dead. That was 56%—10 times the normal rate for hantaviruses in Asia. This disease was a killer.

In the second half of 1993, nearly half of the confirmed cases of hantavirus pulmonary syndrome were fatal. Earlier in the year, though, two-thirds of the patients had died, so even half was an improvement. There were several reasons for the drop in mortality. Physicians were recognizing the disease more quickly and were probably diagnosing less severe cases that had previously been overlooked. They were slowly but surely learning to treat the symptoms of the disease.

WITHIN SIGHT OF THE ENEMY

Meanwhile, researchers were learning more about the virus itself. Antibodies to the virus had been found. The proteins that make up the virus had been found. The genes of the virus had been found, but what of the virus itself?

Actually coaxing a new virus to grow is not easy. During the summer and fall of 1993 teams at both the Centers for Disease Control and the United States Army Medical Research Institute of Infectious Disease at Fort Detrick, Maryland, used a range of laboratory animals and of cells growing in plastic flasks. They were trying to grow the virus from specimens brought from the outbreak region. It wasn't easy. In fact, it was very difficult indeed.

It was known that hantaviruses grow better in samples taken from animals than from humans. The work concentrated on those, specifically, on samples from infected deer mice.

The first genetic information had been obtained at the CDC using materials from USAMRIID, supplied in a spirit of cooperation, but now a race developed between the two. Unfortunately, both thought they had "won," which led to a rivalry that benefited no one. Eventually they agreed to a joint announcement at a meeting in Atlanta on November 3, 1993.

Both had grown the virus in the same kind of cells originally taken from monkey kidneys, and both had grown it from samples taken from deer mice. The CDC used a sample of lung from one of the animals captured in their program earlier in the year, whereas the USAMRIID team, under Dr. Connie Schmaljohn, used a sample from a deer mouse captured near the home of an HPS victim near Convict Creek in California.

Actually growing a virus used to be the definitive test, but with the genetic methods available to the researchers looking at the new hantavirus, they already knew that it had the genes that marked it as a hantavirus. Looking at it using a high-powered electron microscope, they saw exactly what they had expected to see: a hantavirus.

Growing a virus can allow laboratories to produce large amounts of the proteins that make up the virus to use in diagnosis and testing. However, some viruses are just not happy growing outside their normal host, and the new hantavirus turned out to be one of those. It could be grown, but not easily or well. In order to get enough of the proteins to use, researchers had to copy the genes into an easily grown bacterial cell, which would then make large quantities of the viral protein. So growing the virus was not the step forward that had been hoped for.

Now there was a new, small detail to handle, one that was to occupy far more time than it might have taken. Finding a name.

NAMING A DISEASE

When cases began to be seen early in 1993, it was called "an outbreak of acute illness." For a while, when the symptoms were known, it was "unexplained adult respiratory distress syndrome." Then a hantavirus was identified, and it became "hantavirus-associated adult respiratory distress syndrome." Finally, on August 5, 1993, the CDC had given it a new name: hantavirus pulmonary syndrome (HPS).

Now there were two types of hantavirus disease: HFRS in Asia and Europe, and HPS in America.

AND A VIRUS WITHOUT A NAME

As mentioned earlier, there is a whole set of rules that apply to the naming of a virus. They require the name to be in a kind of modernized pseudo-Latin, mostly so that they sound like other scientific names. Virology is new to the naming game and tries to be as "correct" as possible.

The new virus had already been placed in the family *Bunyaviridae,* genus *Hantavirus.* A family is a large grouping, in this case covering everything from the new virus to Rift Valley fever virus in Africa. A genus is a small group of closely related viruses, in the case of genus *Hantavirus,* containing the new virus, as well as Hantaan and Seoul from Asia, Puumala from Europe, and Prospect Hill from America.

What to call the new virus itself?

It is not permitted to name viruses after people and it is difficult to understand why anyone might want the honor. However, some, seeking immortality for themselves or revenge against others, apparently did and so that practice was banned. It is fairly common to name them after the place where they were found, but even this is not always acceptable.

As Dr. C. J. Peters of the CDC noted in his book "Virus Hunter," many people do not want the name of their town immortalized as belonging to a deadly disease, so the name selected is often of some geographical feature, such as a river. There are not that many rivers in the desert.

The first name suggested was "Four Corners virus." It was, after all, a virus that had been found in the Four Corners. That was unacceptable for many reasons. The Navajo Nation objected because the Four Corners Monument is an attraction administered by, and beneficial for, the Navajo.

The Navajo, logically, did not want to be associated with the disease in any way. Studies would show that genetically, risk patterns were not neatly divided along racial lines. By virtue of that first cluster of cases, however, HPS had quickly become known as an "Indian disease" to non-Indians who, at that time, had no better weapons against the disease than denial. By the time the first Anglo cases had been identified in early summer, they already did not want to be publicly identified because HPS was already associated in the widespread perception with "poverty and unsanitary living conditions," the state of affairs that many had managed to convince themselves existed on the reservation.

Many parts of that unfortunate characterization showed a high level of intolerance and ignorance. The Navajo Nation was well ahead of the rest of the country in dealing with this hantavirus, but no one had any illusions that the prejudices would disappear. In that regard, all the Navajo could do was attempt to avoid direct association with the disease that had started out being called "Navajo flu."

Other residents of the Four Corners would have been no more pleased with the name, had they been consulted. The name "Four Corners virus" would have had negative connotations for four states, as well as for a region economically dependent on its ability to attract visitors.

Clearly, that was not a good idea. Next?

The next suggestion was "Muerto Canyon virus," after an arroyo near the site of the first recognized cases. Again, the Navajo had a reason to object. The Navajo are very reverent in speaking about death (*muerto*); they are also mindful that to speak of anything helps to make it happen. Using a phrase with which they were uncomfortable would also have made it very difficult to talk with the Navajo about the disease, and conversation is necessary in order for prevention, diagnosis, and treatment. "Muerto Canyon" was a particularly bad idea, and there was another reason.

The spectacularly beautiful Canyon de Chelly National Monument in Arizona is a place of great importance to the Navajo. Joining with Canyon de Chelly in the National Monument is Cañon del Muerto, the Canyon of Death, named after the massacre of more than a hundred Navajo by Spanish troops in 1805. To commemorate that event with a lethal virus was to add insult to injury.

Maybe it was time to try a river. The name "Convict Creek virus" was vetoed by CDC personnel themselves. After all, although the virus had indeed been grown from a deer mouse captured at Convict Creek, this was from the USAMRIID work, and the CDC did not like that idea, given the dominant role of the CDC in the early work.

This was getting beyond a joke.

The story told of the final naming of the new hantavirus is that scientists were looking through a book of canyons in New Mexico when they found one in about the right area, with a name that they thought nobody could object to: Sin Nombre. Without Name. That is the story, and nobody did object. The name was accepted. Sin Nombre virus it is.

However, that is not quite the whole story. Nobody else has ever managed to find Sin Nombre canyon listed on a map, anywhere. There are quite a few places called "No Name," including a rest area on I-70 through the Colorado Rockies west of Denver, but there is no Sin Nombre to be found.

SIN NOMBRE

There are, in the western United States, many places without names, although they could perhaps more accurately be consid-

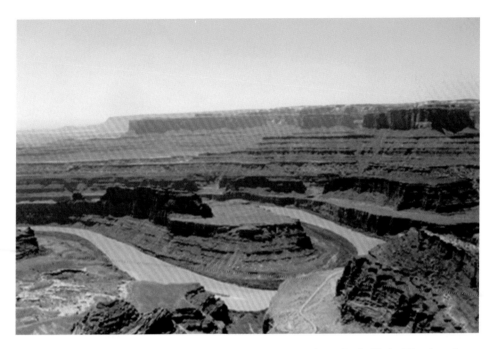

The canyon of the Colorado River from Dead Horse Point State Park, Utah. The river flows 2000 feet below the level of the park. It has taken 150 million years to wear away the rock down to its current level, and it is still eroding it today. As it erodes still further the gigantic canyons of its course, the color of the water changes with the different rocks it passes over. Further down its 1400 mile length, as it passes through Arizona, it erodes still further the Grand Canyon.

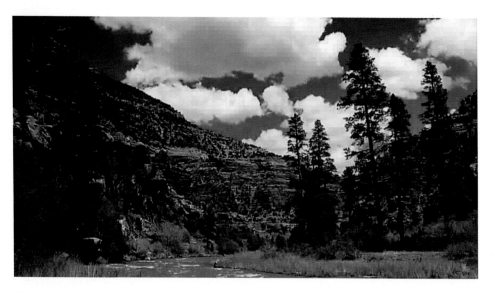

The canyon of the Dolores River in Colorado. The river passing beside crumbling cliffs shows how much time has passed to erode away the millions upon millions of tons of rock that once filled the vastness of the canyon. Each speck of eroded rock coloring the flowing water as it is carried downstream enlarges the canyon by that same minuscule amount. As always in the desert, life gathers around the flow. Plants spring up and then animals congregate. Human settlement of the southwest is also directed by the availability of water, which brings people and animals, including virus-bearing mice, into contact.

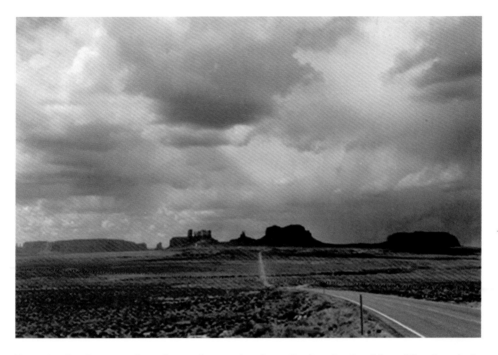

Deep in the desert, red sandstone buttes rise sheer for hundreds of feet. The dry winds scour the rock, rounding corners over the millennia in this supremely dry remnant of a former sea.

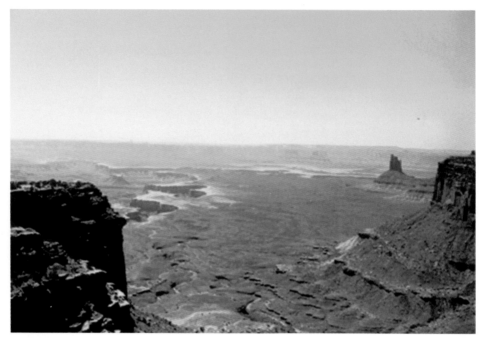

Distance is different when confronted with the huge panoramas of the West. A view from Canyonlands National Park, Utah.

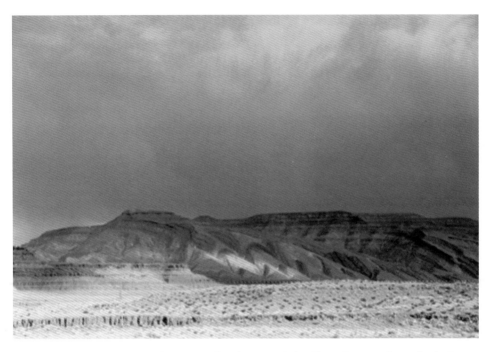

The true nature of the landscape in the deserts of the Four Corners is geological, not biological. Colors come from eons-old sediments rather than the greens of life, which huddles low against the extremes of the desert. Convulsions in the distant past have twisted the rock, lifting the strata to new angles.

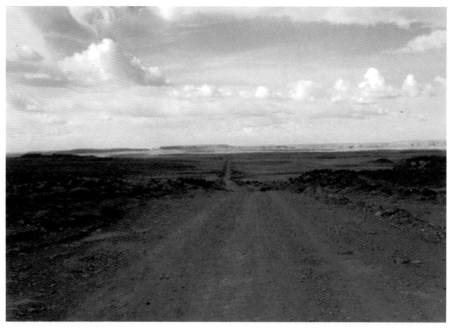

The vast distances and elemental loneliness of much of the Four Corners: an empty desert road close to Chaco Canyon, New Mexico, stretching northward to a distant horizon.

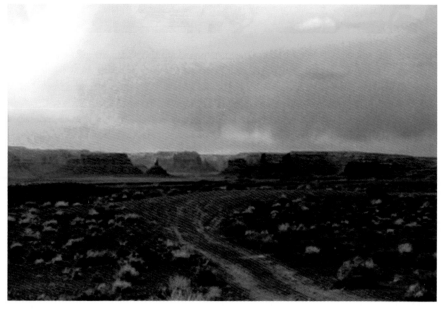

A road winding off into emptiness of sagebrush and distant buttes. The desert contains distances greater than those that meet the eye, and under the sameness lies diversity and complexity.

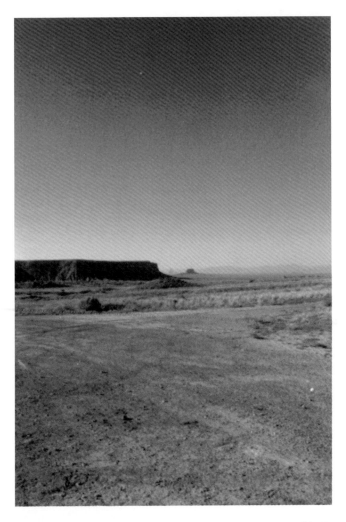

A brilliant blue sky above ocher and dun land. Remote bluffs rising from the parched desert floor and distances draw the eye outward to infinity. This popular image of the Four Corners is like all other generalizations, true only in part, but there are some parts, like this, where they are very true indeed.

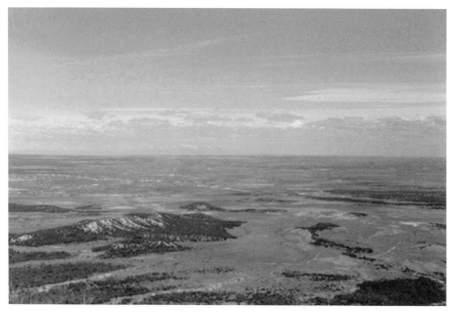

Even where there is the green of life in the uplands of the Four Corners, the land still stretches off into fading blue distances.

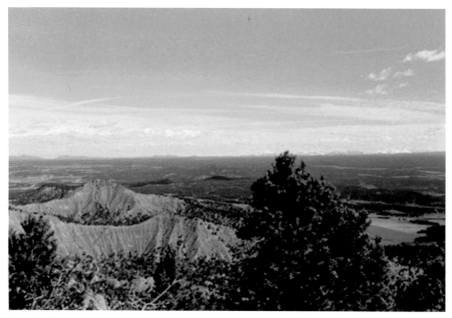

The bluffs of Mesa Verde, overlooking the green uplands of Colorado. Mesa Verde National Park contains the most extensive range of Puebloan cliff dwellings in the United States.

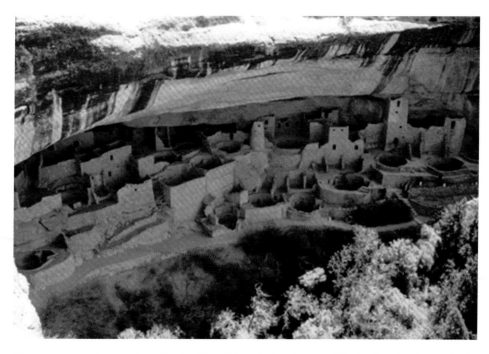

The crowning glory of Mesa Verde, Cliff Palace is the largest cliff dwelling in the world. It was built by the ancestral Puebloans and contains hundreds of rooms (the exact number is still in dispute, but 217 is a widely accepted number). It was home to several hundred people. The round structures at the front of the ruin are *kivas*, of which there are a total of 23. Kivas are underground ceremonial or religious structures; in the floor of each is a small hole, a *sipapu*, symbolizing emergence into the upper world. Steep cliff paths lead to the mesa top where the Puebloans grew maize, beans, and squash using a complex series of dams and pools to gather the infrequent rains. Cliff Palace was built between 1200 and 1274 A.D.; when it was deserted, the inhabitants moved south to the pueblos of New Mexico and Arizona. Why they deserted these huge complexes is still unknown.

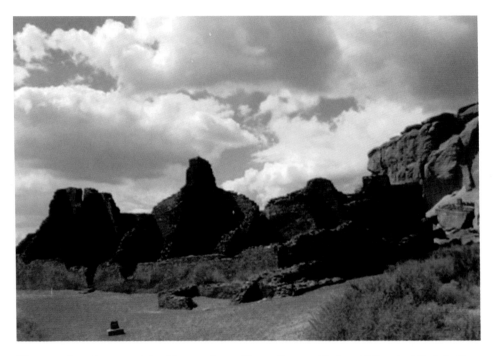

The complex of ancestral Puebloan ruins at Chaco Canyon National Historical Park in New Mexico is the most extensive in the United States. Built on the floor of a shallow canyon, the 13 major villages and "great houses" of Chaco were the center of a trading empire covering thousands of square miles. As with the ruins at Mesa Verde, they were deserted by the builders, although at Chaco this happened earlier, around 1200 A.D.

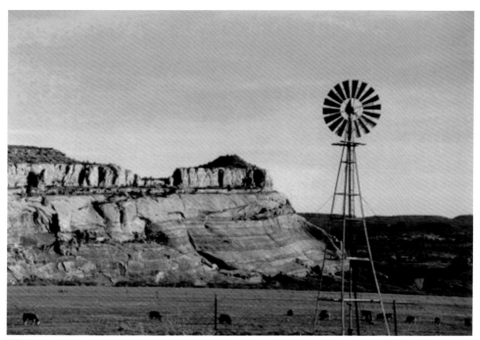

Not all of the Four Corners is arid desert. The deserts of the West can be abundantly fertile in the places where water is available, and a windmill bringing water to the surface can raise lush grass for cattle to graze.

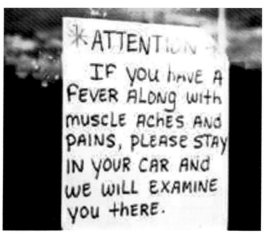

Reaction to the new disease was fueled by the unknown. It was a killer, but in the early days of the outbreak, no one knew how the new disease might be contracted. Because it killed many of those it struck, health-care providers were cautious about exposing other people to suspected victims. No one wanted to turn a health-care facility into an incubator for a deadly disease.

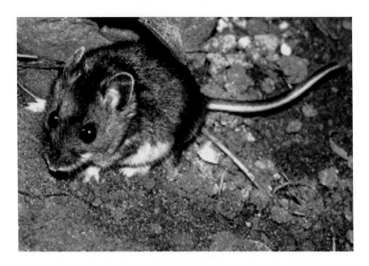

The deer mouse (*Peromyscus maniculatus*). There are three big problems associated with identifying the deer mouse as the source of a virus causing deadly disease. The first is that it lives across a huge range of North America, including most of the United States and much of Canada up to the Yukon; therefore, the virus it hosts is not restricted to a small area. The second is that it is not shy and will happily enter buildings in search of food, exposing people to the virus it carries. The third is that it's cute. It has big eyes and big, rounded ears, with red-brown-gray fur on top and white underneath. Its tail is also lighter underneath. It is 4–8 inches long overall, half of that tail. Deer mice are found in almost any environment, particularly coniferous woodland and scrub. In deer mice, pregnancy produces 4 or 5 kits on average, although there can be up to 10. Pregnancy lasts 3 to 4 weeks. The young are ready to breed when they are 5 weeks old. There are usually three breeding cycles a year, but a warm winter and early spring can add in an extra one, doubling the number of mice that can be produced in that year. Despite their image, deer mice are genuinely frightening. They carry Sin Nombre hantavirus, responsible for 190 out of 196 cases of hantavirus pulmonary syndrome identified in the United States. A subspecies found in Virginia carries Monongahela hantavirus.

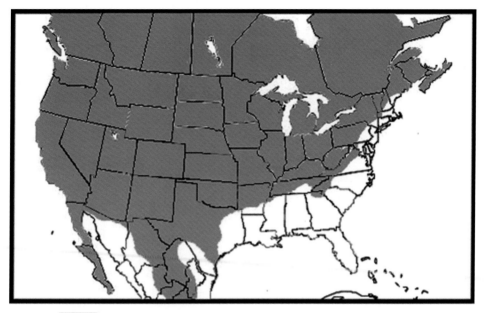

Range of the deer mouse *(Peromyscus maniculatus)*

The deer mouse is found in most areas of the United States, with the exception of the southeast and eastern seaboard. Its range also extends into Mexico and Canada, all the way up to the Yukon and the northwest territory. It shares the southern areas of its range with several related *Peromyscus* mice, but these do not extend into the northern areas.

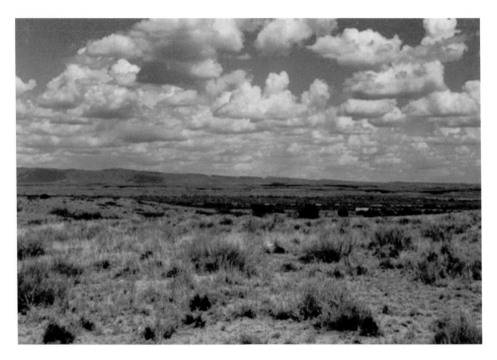

Sixty miles south of Albuquerque, in central New Mexico, is the Sevilleta National Wildlife Refuge. It covers approximately 220,000 acres, spanning the width of the Rio Grande valley and the mountain ranges to either side; the Los Pinos Mountains (pictured) to the east and the Sierra Ladrones to the west. The Rio Grande, the railroad, and Interstate 25 run down the center, which can be seen in the photograph. When long-term ecological research (LTER) programs were created in order to obtain basic information about the American environment, the Sevilleta was an obvious choice. It is situated at the junction of three different ecosystems: Running in from the northwest is a high plateau, growing brush and sagebrush. In the south of the refuge is the Chihuahan desert, studded with creosote bush, which is the terrain type in the picture. To the east is the edge of the Great Plains shortgrass prairie. The Sevilleta LTER program has been operating since 1988 and provided most of the data on mouse numbers during the 1993 hantavirus outbreak.

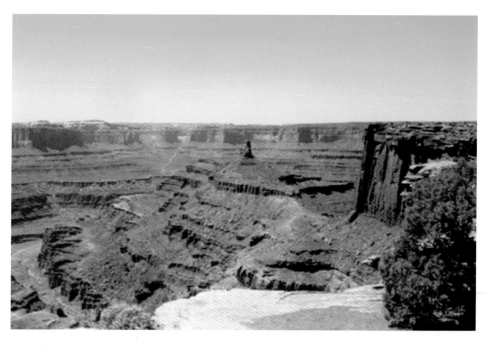

As well as research at the Sevilleta site, rodent numbers were also being studied in Utah. Researchers working in the spectacularly beautiful scenery of Canyonlands National Park were able to supply long-term data on rodent numbers to the 1993 investigation. Sadly, the Utah study was cut short when dangers of handling rodents became apparent. Although Canyonlands is a harsh place, even among the stark, eroded cliffs some plants manage to scratch a precarious living. The ledge in the foreground is "slickrock," an unfamiliar term to those accustomed to lusher climes, but one that appropriately describes the bare rock with occasional pools of forming soil that top the sandstone buttes and mesas.

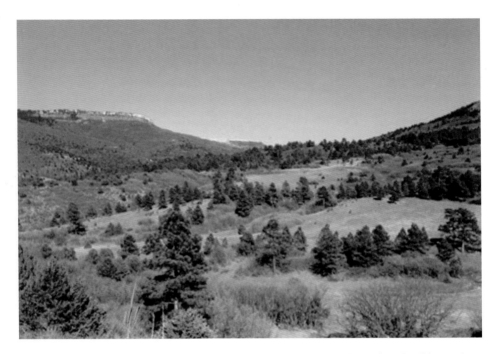

In the fall of 1993 there was enormous concern about a possible outbreak of hantavirus disease in the fall. There was huge relief when data were collected showing that mouse numbers were actually falling. That work was carried out among the alpine meadows of Pecos National Monument north of Santa Fe, New Mexico, shown here. The trees are piñon pines and junipers. This is typical upland habitat, of the type favored by deer mice.

ered spaces. There are more places with several names: Native American names from various and even multiple tribes, Spanish names, Anglo names, and local colloquial names. Many of the older names are forgotten, or at least unspoken. No one knows what the ancestral Puebloans called Chaco Canyon, Muerto Canyon, or the vast reaches still without names.

The official naming of the virus as "no name" is a pointed comment to all the people who would not let it be named after anything they had an interest in, but it is also strangely appropriate.

Sin Nombre virus. The virus without a name. The mysterious killer that came to town.

The killer might not have a name, but it had a family.

7

HANTAVIRUSES: OUT OF ASIA

· ·

All armies prefer high ground to low and sunny ground to shady. If an army occupies high ground . . . it will not suffer countless diseases.
> GENERAL SUN TZU, *The Art of War,* 500 B.C.
> Kingdom of Wu in what is now Jiangsu Province, northern China

· ·

But there is neither East nor West, Border, nor Breed, nor Birth
> RUDYARD KIPLING, *The Ballad of East and West,* 1889

· ·

As the ecological research was being conducted in the Four Corners in the hope of learning how to prevent human cases of the disease, attention among the medical researchers was focused on what was known about other hantaviruses. Somewhat ironically, hantaviruses had first been brought to the official attention of the United States government because of its military presence in another sovereign nation far from the Navajo reservation.

KOREA

At 4 A.M. on June 25, 1950, an artillery barrage heralded the invasion of South Korea by troops of the North Korean Army. When the forces of "Great Leader" Kim Il Sung crossed the border, they met little effective resistance.

For hundreds of years an isolated land caught between China and Japan, Korea fell under Japanese influence late in the 19th century. Korea had been a Japanese protectorate for 40 years when the end of World War II brought the collapse of the Japanese occupation. The victorious Red Army, surging south through Manchuria in August 1945, stopped at a paper line, defined in Washington, approximately halfway down the Korean peninsula: the 38th parallel. This became the border between two new states: communist North Korea, with close ties to China and to the Soviet Union, and the American-dominated South Korea.

Relations between the divided nations were never easy, but when, after years of military clashes, the 135,000-strong North Korean army invaded in full strength, it seemed unstoppable. While in numbers the 95,000-strong South Korean army was not badly outmatched, in training and equipment it was hopelessly outclassed. As a matter of policy, America had not given the South Korean military heavy weapons or combat aircraft. This made the attack aircraft and battle tanks of the North Korean Army almost invincible.

North Korean forces took the South Korean capital, Seoul, in 2 days, on the same day that the United Nations, meeting in New York, resolved to repel the aggressors. Forces from the United States and the British Commonwealth were to provide the main firepower behind this resolution, although eventually troops from more than 20 countries would become involved.

The first U.S. ground troops landed in Korea from occupied Japan on July 1, but proved unable to halt the North Korean advance. Within the month, all South Korean and United Nations forces were driven back to a small area of land in the southeastern corner of the country around the port of Pusan, the "Pusan Perimeter." Here, the North Korean advance was checked, and the steady buildup of U.N. military power continued.

On September 15, 1950, the U.S. Marines staged amphibious landings at Inchon near Seoul. A day later, U.N. forces broke out of the Pusan Perimeter and began to drive north. The combination of firepower and airpower proved devastating. Seoul was retaken within 2 weeks, and on October 25, South Korean forces reached the Yalu River, which formed the northern border between North Korea and China.

The Chinese had threatened repeatedly that such a northward drive would bring them into the war. It did. Chinese forces first entered combat at the beginning of November. The Chinese army at the time contained five million men, and this intervention once more turned the tide of the war. Seoul was evacuated on January 4, 1951, and was held by Chinese forces until March 14, when it was retaken by U.N. forces heading north once more.

This sweeping war, moving from one end of the Korean peninsula to the other, crossing and recrossing the 38th parallel and the nearby Hantaan River, became much less mobile at the end of June as the two sides dug in. On July 10, the two sides began talking at Kaesong. Despite this, the war carried on for 2 more years, until July 12, 1953. After all the suffering and the deaths of millions, the new border was very close to the 38th parallel.

Korea was the first military confrontation between the new superpowers, but as in all such wars, stand-ins were used, and direct Soviet involvement was only admitted many years later. In the skies above Korea, the latest technology went head to head, with the first combats between the new jet fighters catching the public eye. On the ground, though, the lot of the infantryman was, as ever, mud and blood.

Total casualties in the war are still unknown. Of the United Nations forces, 37,000 died, along with 415,000 South Korean troops. Casualty figures from the Chinese and North Korean forces are unavailable, but estimates of a million dead are common. While these were the casualties among soldiers, as with any "modern" war, many civilians were also killed.

Many of the casualties died not from enemy fire, but from the other riders of the apocalypse, famine and pestilence. The spread of diseases served to fuel persistent rumors of biological warfare during the Korean War, which gained momentum from a variety of sources. At one point a dead mouse wearing a parachute was discovered deep in Chinese-held territory. This later turned out to be an example of very black humor by U.N. prisoners of war, although they could not have known how prophetic it was.

THE TRENCH WAR

From July 1951 to 1953, the front line was more like that in the trenches of World War I. Even Field Marshal Lord Alexander, a British veteran of the World War I, commented on the similarity. Heavily entrenched forces faced each other across fiercely defended "no-man's land" as they dug ever deeper into the stony ground. Battles were for a single hill rather than a whole country.

Despite fierce attacks and huge loss of life the front line moved no more than a few miles in those 2 years. As the soldiers in Flanders had discovered many years before, with life in the trenches came misery, sickness, and death. In Flanders, "trench nephritis" was a mysterious disease, causing several thousand casualties. Many years before, during the American Civil War, yet another "trench war," 14,000 cases of a similar disease had been seen in Union forces in the central sector. The cause of these diseases remained unknown. It was in Korea that it was finally to come to light.

KOREAN HEMORRHAGIC FEVER

In the summer of 1951, U.N. troops began to fall sick with a lethal new disease. It started with fevers and muscle pains, and in two-thirds or more of cases, recovery followed with the whole disease looking like a case of influenza. In the others, however, the disease ran its full, deadly course.

After a few days of fever, the characteristic blood-filled small hemorrhages known as *petechiae* began to appear across the skin, showing that the cells of the blood vessels themselves were under attack by the most deadly of human diseases, hemorrhagic fever. As blood began to leak from damaged vessels, blood pressure fell dramatically and shock often set in. Inside the body, the kidneys began to disintegrate, with the cells lining the tiny tubes that filter the blood dying and falling away, blocking more of the kidney as they did so. Parts of the kidney began to die. Then, as the kidneys failed, blood pressure rose and, combined with the hemorrhages spread throughout the body, blood seeped into the body and the brain.

Of the patients who developed these symptoms, up to half would die. Those who survived would experience a convalescence lasting months as their kidneys slowly began to function again.

The speed and severity of this disease brought it to the attention of doctors with the U.N. forces. At first, many possible causes were suspected, ranging from cancer to smallpox, but the pattern of disease convinced them that they were dealing with a new infection, which they named "Korean hemorrhagic fever." By the end of the war, it had struck down over 3200 U.N.

troops. More than 2500 of them were Americans, and of these 121 were to die. The disease also hit unknown numbers of allied and opposing military and civilian personnel. United Nations cases were evacuated by helicopter to a special facility near Uijonbu for intensive study and treatment, but the cause was to prove difficult to find.

Observations in the field and some of the experimental work had provided good evidence that the virus was spread by contact with rodents, either directly or by their droppings and urine, but there was no identification of the cause.

Although this disease was unfamiliar to western doctors, this was not the first time it had been seen.

LESSONS FROM HISTORY

Although this disease was new to western medicine, it had been observed before. There is a description of a disease with similar symptoms in a Chinese medical book, "Whang-Jae-Nae-Kyung," dating from 960 A.D., almost a thousand years earlier. With the development of modern investigative medicine, multiple reports started coming in of a similar disease.

The border between Russia and China is formed for much of its length by the valley of the Amur and Ussuri Rivers. The Amur is one of the world's great rivers, running for 3000 miles, and is over 10 miles wide at its mouth. The land around the river has long been a source of conflict. Treaties signed in the 19th century between Tsarist Russia and Imperial China established the current border, but even now there is still conflict.

Although cases had been observed since 1913, it was in 1932 that doctors in the Soviet Union (as it was then) reported a similar disease in the lower Amur valley, calling it by a variety of names: Churilov's disease, Far Eastern nephroso-nephritis, hemorrhagic nephroso-nephritis, or hemorrhagic fever with renal syndrome. They also linked the disease with exposure to rodents, but lacked the technology to follow the link any further.

The disease was seen across the border as well. Manchuria is the region of northeastern China that borders both on Korea and on the Amur River valley. In the years leading up to World War II, up to a million Japanese troops were stationed in Manchuria to support the "independent" puppet state of Manchukuo, established in 1932 and "ruled" by the last Chinese emperor, P'u-i. Among these troops, 12,000 cases of a similar disease were seen. Here, it was called by yet more names; Songo fever, Tayinshan disease, Nidoko fever, or epidemic hemorrhagic fever (EHF). This was only part of the range of the disease in China, where more than 20,000 cases were reported each year after it was identified in 1931.

From among the many names the disease had gathered throughout history, it was the Russian name that was to stick: hemorrhagic fever with renal syndrome.

THEN AND NOW

In South Korea, following the end of the war in 1953, the disease appeared in civilians moving back into the demilitarized zone around the new border. It took several years to establish itself, causing 20 cases in 1955. Since then the disease has spread slowly southwest from its original focus around the cease-fire line, and the number of cases has stabilized at 300 to 900 a year. Little information has come out of the closed society of North Korea, but from what has emerged it is clear that the virus has spread in both directions.

The death rate from Hantaan infection in South Korea has been reduced to approximately 5% overall, which seems to be the same among rural Korean villagers and U.S. military personnel, despite the differences in medical care.

China remains the major focus of the disease. It has been estimated that at least 40,000 to 100,000 cases occur every year, and the number of cases is increasing. From 1950 to 1995, there have been 1,169,570 officially reported cases of HFRS with 43,458 deaths, a mortality rate of 3.72%. Not all of these were caused by Hantaan virus, and the other viruses responsible for HFRS are detailed later on. Although the numbers in individual provinces are extremely variable from year to year, 28 out of 31 Chinese provinces are known to have HFRS present.

In a large study of risk factors for hantavirus infection in China, the main factor was, as expected, activities likely to increase contact with rodents. These included extended working on farms and living in accommodation in fields or at the edge of villages. Straw piles near houses are common in rural China, and these also seemed to increase the risk of disease, probably by providing homes for rodents close to those of humans. One surprising finding was that ownership of a cat increased risk. Villagers in China often keep cats to control rodents, and while the virus has been isolated from a cat, it is not known if they can infect humans directly. While "outside" predators such as coyotes, owls, or barn cats may be protective, house cats often bring prey into the house to play with it, which is probably a significant route of exposure for the owners.

Better understanding of the course of HFRS has reduced the number who die, and other viruses are less lethal, but Hantaan HFRS still kills 5–10 out of every hundred cases, and in some outbreaks, up to 20 in a hundred will die. It is a huge problem in China, and a current one. In September 1998, as huge floods in the area began to recede, the health department of Heilonjiang Province in northeastern China issued an emergency circular noting concern over increased numbers of rodents and warning of a possible HFRS epidemic.

VARIATIONS IN A VIRUS

The time from exposure to Hantaan virus to the development of symptoms seems to vary widely, with an average of 10 to 25 days, but sometimes varying from 1 to 6 weeks. Why this varies so widely is not known, but it may be related to differences between individuals as much as the nature of the infection.

Hantaan seems to be a classic zoonosis, a disease spread directly from animals to humans with no or almost no spread between infected individuals. There does seem to be at least the possibility of transmission from mother to child, but this is very rare, with only one documented case of infection of the fetus.

Like most virus diseases, HFRS does not occur evenly throughout the year. There is a small peak in the number of infections at the end of spring, but the main peak is later. In a major Korean study covering the years 1966–1986, over half of all cases occurred in the last 3 months of the year, with over a third in November alone. This pattern of increases lags slightly behind similar changes in the number of rodents in these areas, another factor in linking the disease to the rodents.

In areas of Korea where the infection is established (endemic), almost 4% of the population have antibodies to the virus, showing that they have been infected at some time. Away from these areas, the rate drops to 1%, but the disease does not affect all people equally. There is a link to rural workers, often farmers or soldiers in rural locations, especially around the focus of the disease on the cease-fire line. The disease occurs mostly in those aged between 20 and 50 years old, although there are a few mild cases in young children.

We now know that the ratio of male and female rodents infected with hantaviruses is different in different species, and differences in behavior may be responsible. There is a link to gender in humans as well. In Korea, HFRS cases in men outnumber those in women by two or three to one.

FINDING HANTAAN

Although the cause had not been identified, it was clear that this was an infectious disease. Early in the 1940s, Soviet scientists injected blood and urine from patients with the disease into "volunteers." This was at the high point of Stalin's reign, and it is likely that the term "volunteer" was quite flexibly interpreted. Whatever the methods, it was established that the subjects did become sick with the same symptoms. One experiment showed that the infectious agent could pass a fine filter that would stop bacteria. This method has been used since 1892 to identify virus diseases. HFRS seemed to be caused by a virus.

In related work, Japanese doctors reported that similar experiments with monkeys produced the disease and that extracts of parasites from field mice could produce the same effect. However, no other workers have been able to produce the disease in monkeys, despite extensive efforts, and it has been suggested that the real subjects of these experiments were unwilling humans. Horrific as it seems, this is possible.

Under the Japanese warrior ethic, termed *Bushi-do* ("the way of the warrior"), it is the duty of the defeated soldier to die fighting. Surrender is the loss of all honor, so any soldier who surrendered was, to the Japanese, beneath contempt and classed as subhuman. To European or American troops, surrender was an acceptable part of war and prisoners were required to be well treated. Indeed, conditions governing the humane treatment of prisoners of war were laid down in the western version of the "rules of war," the Geneva Conventions. So defeated Allied troops surrendered, and from this clash of cultures came many horrors.

One of the worst was Unit 731, operating out of a prison camp in occupied Manchuria. This was a specialist "research" medical unit that performed a range of lethal "tests" on human subjects selected from the ranks of the prisoners taken by Japanese forces. The subjects died of exposure, poisoning, and disease, any subject deemed worthy of such "investigation." In such a setting, testing a threatening disease on these subjects would seem quite normal.

Fortunately, more acceptable approaches to virology were eventually able to identify the cause of the disease.

In 1976, Professor Ho Wang Lee and his group at Korea University in Seoul collected samples of rodents from the affected areas. Studying these, they showed a novel protein in the lungs of Asian striped field mice (*Apodemus agrarius*) that reacted with blood from patients recovering from HFRS. The virus is also found in other hosts, but this apparently insignificant mouse seems to be the main source of the virus that caused so much suffering and which required so much effort to find. Two years later, Lee's group showed that this protein was from the agent that caused the disease, which could be grown in the type of field mice it had first been isolated from. The protein was found in many organs inside the mouse for over 2 months at high levels, particularly the lungs, and reacted with blood from patients with the disease. Strangely, it did not seem to harm the mouse.

It had already been shown that Hantaan infection of humans matched variations in the number of mice. Professor Lee's team also showed that the proportion of mice carrying the virus varied in the same way, with the same two peaks over the course of the year. In the winter, so few mice had the virus that of the 85 mice tested, the virus was not detected in any of them. In the spring, however, the virus was found in up to 16% of mice and in the fall that more than doubled to 37%. Yet another link had been discovered between infection of mice and human disease. The cause of HFRS in Korea had been found.

Because Lee had found the virus in mice captured near the Hantaan River, close to the 38th parallel and the town of Songnaeri, it was called Hantaan virus. As the "virus hunter" C. J. Peters has noted, naming unpleasant viruses after rivers offends fewer people than naming them after towns.

Later work managed to identify cells in which the virus could grow, allowing it to be grown in flasks in the laboratory.

Although the virus cannot be grown in monkeys, the cells used are derived from an African monkey, but these isolated, *cultured* cells are very different to the whole host animal, a fact that often is forgotten.

By using different filters, the agent was shown to be about 0.000075 mm (75 nm) across, about average for a virus. It was destroyed by detergent or ether, showing it had an outer coat of fatty membrane from the host cell. In 1982, using an electron microscope, which can see down to where the waves of light itself are too long to be of any use, a virus was seen. When the genes of the virus were extracted, they were found to be made of ribonucleic acid in three unequal parts, looking like those seen in viruses belonging to a family called Bunyaviridae, which contains many viruses threatening to humans.

The identification of Hantaan also allowed the identification of other hantaviruses, as antibodies to Hantaan were able to detect the proteins of related viruses. In addition, the proteins of the virus itself could be used to examine blood from patients with diseases thought to be other types of HFRS.

There was another use for these proteins. In 1990, 600 stored blood samples from 245 patients who had contracted HFRS during the Korean War were tested. All but 15 showed antibodies against the virus. Here was further proof that Hantaan had been the culprit then.

Carleton Gajdusek, who won the Nobel Prize for Medicine in 1976 for his work on destructive brain diseases and also had a long-standing interest in this area, reviewed the findings of Ho Wang Lee's group and identified 52 separate areas across Europe and Asia where similar diseases have been observed. He also noted that a number of infections caused by other viruses had been included in the general classification of "epidemic hemorrhagic fever." He suggested that the real grouping was of the hemorrhagic fevers with kidney damage originating from rodents, and that across the whole supercontinent of Europe and Asia they were closely related. He proposed that they should be renamed to reflect their origin, as "muroid virus ne-phropathies," but the name HFRS was to stick. It is hard to change a name once it is given.

HANTAVIRUSES

In 1985 the genus *Hantavirus* was formally defined. This group-ing, above species and below family, is a working classification for similar groups of viruses. Species cannot really be defined for viruses, but it does not stop people from trying and from imposing all of the other Latin-sounding structures of the for-mal *Linnaean* naming system: genus, family, order, and so on. Because mankind has a driving need to put things into order, hantaviruses were placed in the family *Bunyaviridae*, cousins to viruses such as the deadly African Rift Valley fever, which was in the genus *Phlebovirus* within the *Bunyaviridae*.

While the hantaviruses closely resemble the other bunyavi-ruses in size, structure, and the way their genes are organized, there are important differences. Although viruses in this family usually grow in animals and are then passed on to humans, most of them are passed by insects and mites, acting as "vectors" for the infection (see Chapter 10). Of the bunyaviruses, it is only the hantaviruses that do not seem able to use this route. As far as humans are concerned, this seems to be a very good thing, as it reduces the chances of becoming infected. Other members of the family are passed in this way, and kill.

Why hantaviruses cannot be spread by insects is a mystery. Although the idea of insects spreading HFRS or even hantavirus pulmonary syndrome is worrisome, it seems unlikely that they will acquire this ability easily. Individual hantaviruses are very well adapted to their rodent hosts and show every sign of having been coexisting with them for millions of years. The hantavirus expert Dr. Charles Calisher has suggested that they may repre-sent living fossils, from the days before bunyaviruses acquired the ability to spread by insects or mites. Surviving so successfully in their particular rodent host, they have had no impetus to evolve further and acquire the ability to spread by such a route.

Hantaviruses are only spread directly by body fluids and excretions of the infected rodent. This is not to say that they cannot infect other hosts. They can. One type, however, seems to provide the virus with a long-term home, and in that host, the virus does not kill. It grows and infectious virus is released, at least for several months, and possibly for the whole life of the rodent host, without causing any apparent disease or any other than minor effects, such as a raised number of white cells in the blood of the mouse. In humans, the story can be very different.

TOWN HANTAVIRUS

Seoul is the capital city of the Republic of (South) Korea. It is one of the world's megacities, with a population of over 10 million, and is the center of the industrial tiger that South Korea has become. Anything further from the rice paddies and granaries that field mice like to call home, and that humans had learned to associate with HFRS, is hard to imagine, and yet there were reports of another type of HFRS in Korea. About 100 blood samples per year from Seoul and other Korean cities were testing positive for antibodies to Hantaan virus, and a milder form of HFRS was occurring. Although it was not as deadly, killing one in a hundred, the symptoms were similar to those of Hantaan HFRS. They tend to be shorter and less distinct, with abdominal pain and liver and kidney problems the main features. However, it was very clear that there was a hantavirus loose in Seoul, and it was killing.

Rodents were immediately the prime suspects, and the rodent host for Hantaan was known. However, surveys of rodents around the urban locations where the disease had occurred showed no *Apodemus* mice. This was expected. They are, after all, field mice, and there are few fields in urban Seoul. Unsurprisingly, in an urban area, rats were found. Of 477 brown rats captured in Seoul, 63 had antibody showing past infection and 37 of those even had the proteins of a hantavirus present. Further work showed that the brown rat (*Rattus norvegicus*) and, less often, the black rat (*Rattus rattus*) could act as carriers for the disease. Humans had long known to fear rats as carriers of bubonic plague, but here was yet another disease that they brought to humans.

While antibodies to the new virus reacted with the proteins of Hantaan, showing that it was related, they reacted weakly enough that it was shown as different. In 1985 it was classified as a new hantavirus, named Seoul virus. In this case, it was apparently acceptable to name the virus after a place rather than a river. This was just as well because the river that runs by Seoul is the Han. That could have been confusing.

As with Hantaan, Seoul virus seemed to have been around for some time. In the 1960s, 130 cases of HFRS were seen in urban Osaka, Japan. However, rats are not restricted to towns and neither is Seoul virus. In rural China, it appears that both Hantaan and Seoul viruses are circulating, with Hantaan HFRS outnumbering Seoul HFRS between two and five to one. The symptoms are similar, and Seoul seems to affect mainly adults in the same age range as Hantaan, so they are often not separated as causes of HFRS in such areas. Unlike Hantaan, cases of Seoul HFRS seems to peak once a year from late fall to early spring, possibly reflecting rats spending the winter in houses to keep warm. It is a different disease than Hantaan HFRS, with a different cause.

The World Health Organization recognizes three types of HFRS: rural, as with Hantaan; urban, as with Seoul; and laboratory-acquired HFRS.

HANTAVIRUS AT WORK

Seoul seems to have been responsible for a number of outbreaks of HFRS among laboratory workers. In Korea and Japan, between 1976 and 1987, 33 separate outbreaks produced 164 cases of HFRS, with one death. These infections come from natural Seoul virus infections of the laboratory rat, yet another host for the virus. They also seem to occur mostly in winter, for reasons that are not clear. Other outbreaks of "laboratory" HFRS have been seen in Belgium, the Netherlands (Holland), France, the United Kingdom, Finland, and the Soviet Union. In Moscow in 1962, 83 cases of HFRS were seen. It was these infections in workers who had been exposed to air around the rats that helped identify spread in the air as the main route of infection and the rat as the source.

SEOUL GOES GLOBAL

Seoul-associated HFRS is typically milder than the Hantaan form, but it still kills one of every hundred cases. It is a worrying disease, all the more so for signs in some areas that the severity of Seoul HFRS is increasing. Unlike the Asian yellow-striped field mouse, rats go anywhere that humans go. Many of them had antibody to Seoul virus, all around the world, on every continent except Antarctica.

Seaports are a particular concern for the entry of infected rats. In Taiwan, a major seaport, Seoul seems to be the only hantavirus circulating. In Japan the rate of infection in rodents captured at the port of Hakata in Fukuoka Prefecture has risen from 0.5 to 32% over the 16 years to 1996. In Alexandria, Egypt, 12% of rats have antibody to Seoul, as do 12% of sailors. In the 1996 Belgian outbreak described in more detail later on, 6 of 199 cases appeared actually to be due to Seoul virus. The virus is also in the Americas; it is a global disease.

Unsurprisingly, Americans were concerned about the ability of the virus to cause disease in the United States. A study reported in 1987 concentrated on rats in urban Baltimore. In the words of the scientists who ran the study, "In the alleyways of the inner cities, litter and trash abound." Where there are piles of trash, they observed, there are rats. A hantavirus was found, and although it was rather cautiously named "Baltimore rat virus," it was very similar to Seoul. As with Hantaan, the biggest and oldest rats had the highest levels of antibody; up to 80% were positive for hantavirus.

Johns Hopkins Hospital in Baltimore is one of the world's leading institutions for the study of infectious disease. During 3 years of study, from January 1986 to October 1988, scientists at Johns Hopkins tested patients for kidney damage and antibody to hantavirus. No patients were shown to have current hantavirus disease, and although antibody was detected, only 15 of 1148 patients tested positive for the local hantavirus. In an analysis of the results of the study, a significant link was shown with kidney malfunction linked to high blood pressure in these 15 suggesting that hantavirus could be causing kidney damage inside the United States of America.

After the study was complete, three patients were seen to develop a disease very similar to the mild form of HFRS associated with Seoul virus, during which they developed antibody to the local strain of hantavirus, which seemed increasingly likely to be the American version of Seoul.

The Baltimore study was the first demonstration of HFRS in the Americas since a possible outbreak during the Civil War. If it was a hantavirus that brought so much misery to 14,000 Union troops, it was very probably Seoul, carried by rats in the trenches.

Seoul is still there. During 1996 and 1997, 8 out of 72 rats trapped and tested in Los Angeles were reported to have antibody to Seoul virus.

Experts have questioned the results of both American studies. At the time of the Baltimore study, and up to 1993, it was thought that any hantavirus disease in the Americas would show up as kidney disease. We have since learned it would not.

In 1989, Professor Ho Wang Lee stated of Seoul virus HFRS: "This type threatens to endanger the world as never before." This seemed a very real threat following his finding of human disease resulting from infection with Seoul virus, the host rodent of which lives in close contact with humans with a genuinely worldwide distribution that is almost impossible to eradicate. However, apart from isolated studies like those in Baltimore and Belgium, Seoul virus has not yet been confirmed as a major cause of disease outside eastern Asia.

Again, in the words of Professor Lee, "accumulating evidence suggests that HFRS is misdiagnosed . . . in many parts of the world." The list of possible misidentifications is almost as long as the suggested causes for Hantaan HFRS at Uijonbu, ranging from hepatitis to influenza. Definitive studies have not yet been performed in the teeming port cities where it would have its firmest foothold. Until they are, we cannot relax about this potential danger.

Despite Seoul, concern over hantaviruses in the Americas was soon to be redirected, from the kidneys to the lungs.

8

OTHER HANTAVIRUSES

. . . .

Every one of you has his particular plague.

PITTACUS, FROM PLUTARCH,
Morals, on the Tranquility of the Mind

. . . .

PUUMALA

HFRS has another form, not as damaging, and far from China or Korea. The main focus of the milder, European form of HFRS seems to be in northern Scandinavia, above 60° of latitude. This is a dark, damp land, much of it covered with thick pine forests, but cases have been seen across the whole of Europe, even down to the shores of the Mediterranean Sea.

The European form of HFRS had been suggested to be linked to the Asian cases by Carleton Gadjusek. The clinical definition of the disease was based on seven Swedish cases reported during 1933–1934, the first of which was an 18-year-old girl with kidney disease in the Central Hospital of Östersund. The disease was named nephropathia epidemica (NE, epidemic kidney damage) or sometimes epidemic benign nephropathy (EBN). It was to take almost 50 years to identify the virus that caused it.

NE is far milder than the HFRS caused by Hantaan, but is still a very unpleasant disease, with fever, back pain, headache, and decreased urine production followed by a massive increase. Although the infection damages the kidneys, the hemorrhagic symptoms that are so damaging with Hantaan are rarely seen. The death rate from NE is normally much less than 1% although there are reports of some outbreaks where levels above 5% were seen. In the 1997 outbreak in Bashkortostan, Russia, severe cases were seen at an unusually high rate, although the death rate was still much lower than with Hantaan at 0.35%.

The time between exposure and symptoms appears to be longer than for Hantaan but again shows great variability, ranging from 1 to 8 weeks. Although the disease is less damaging, recovery of full kidney function is not always seen, and long-term increases in blood pressure may also result from infection.

NE is caused by one of the group of Eurasian HFRS viruses and is classified as a rural-type HFRS, but damage to other parts of the body does occur, including the lungs. Shortness of breath is reported, and analysis shows lung damage. Here, one of the classic causes of HFRS was showing some of the signs that were to become so very familiar when hantavirus pulmonary syndrome made its appearance.

In the words of the investigators, "HFRS and HPS may be . . . more similar than appears from the clinical presentations."

As with Hantaan, it took a long time to identify the cause. Again, the first identification was of a part of the virus, using serum from patients recovering from NE. In 1980, this serum was used to identify a protein from the virus in the bank vole, *Clethrionomys glareolus*. Once more, a rodent carried a hantavirus that could transfer to humans and cause disease.

Although voles are less apparent to humans than rats or mice, there are large numbers of them in rural and wooded areas, and they form a major reservoir for disease. There is a clear link between the number of bank voles and the number of NE cases, and the number of rodents in the houses of NE patients is also higher. The bank vole is a country rodent and, as expected, NE is a rural disease. In parallel with HFRS in China, NE has been linked to wood piles close to houses, which could act as homes for the voles in the way that straw piles do for rats and mice in rural China.

Unlike Hantaan HFRS, there is a single peak of NE, with infections highest in the autumn, explained by the movement of bank voles into houses and outbuildings seeking food and shelter from the cold, where they come into closer contact with each other and with humans, or, in the rather odd words of the scientists themselves, "human exposure mainly occurs when bank voles seasonally utilize anthropogenic vole harbourage."

The virus was grown for the first time in 1984 and was named Puumala, after a region of southeastern Finland where it was well established. Puumala has also been shown in related voles and it seems to be able to infect even rats and mice, although whether it can be spread by them is not known.

There is some evidence that the outbreak of NE that caused thousands of cases among German troops stationed in Finland during World War II was spread by lemmings, but it is hard to prove such a claim this long after the event. More recent work has shown antibody to Puumala virus in small numbers of Swedish moose, expanding the possible host animals considerably, although it is unlikely that the virus grows well in so distant a relative of its normal host. At any rate, infestation of a house with moose is unlikely and would be rather visible even if it happened, further reducing any risk.

Puumala-like viruses seem to be present in many regions and in many animals. They are the most likely candidate to have caused the "trench nephritis" of Flanders. They are seen across Europe and well into Asia. The locations where such viruses are found has expanded recently to include, by a strange turn of fate, Korea, where antibody has been found in a range of rodents and also in bats and even birds. But, as usual, it is likely that only a few hosts can pass on the virus. This Puumala-like virus is likely to be a native Korean equivalent of Puumala, possibly the newly identified Muju virus, which infects the main Korean vole species, *Eothenomys regulus*.

NE seems to occur mainly in the same sections of the population as Hantaan and is a major cause of human disease. Although it is (fortunately) less severe than Hantaan or Seoul HFRS, there are many similarities to Hantaan. For NE, most cases occur between the ages of 20 to 50 years, probably causing even milder disease in children. Men are more likely to develop the disease than women, by a ration of from 2:1 to 3.5:1. The people most at risk are those with rural occupations or activities, with hunters and farmers at particular risk.

Most work with Puumala has been done in the Scandinavian countries, particularly at the Universities of Umeå and Helsinki, and in these countries thousands of cases are seen every year. These are mainly in the northern regions, where antibodies to Puumala virus is found in up to 20% of the general population. However, antibodies to Puumala-type hantaviruses appear to be present in 1 to 2% of the population in areas across much of Europe, even as far south as Portugal. In 1996, 199 cases of the mild HFRS typical of NE were seen in Belgium, close to the grass and crops that now grow over the abandoned trenches of Flanders. They came mainly from the forested southern area and were almost all identified as being due to Puumala, with 6 identified as Seoul virus and 11 as a new hantavirus, Dobrava.

OTHER HANTAVIRUSES: DOBRAVA

Greece and the shattered lands that now make up what was once Yugoslavia lie a long way from the dark pine forests of northern Scandinavia. They border on the Mediterranean, a blue, inland sea that is to Europe what the Caribbean is to America. Yet in the mid-1980s, 27 cases of a very severe HFRS were seen, mainly in the late summer. The symptoms were far more like Hantaan than Puumala, but with an even higher fatality rate of 15%. Unlike Hantaan, the lungs seem to be involved, filling with fluid in a way that would become chillingly familiar a few years later.

A virus was grown from one of the patients and, as expected, was found to be a hantavirus. Although it seemed to be related to Hantaan, it was different enough to be classed as yet another new virus.

Again, as with Hantaan, identification of a virus allowed the development of tests, and the virus was found in other countries in that area of southeastern Europe known as the Balkans. In the shattered remnants of Yugoslavia, the same virus was killing up to 20% of cases. This was not surprising given the effects of the war, but was very worrying.

It was in one of the republics formed from what was Yugoslavia that the host was to be found. *Apodemus flavicollis,* the yellow-necked field mouse, inhabits a broad swathe of Europe, mainly in the south, but this particular mouse was captured in Dobrava, Slovenia. Now this virus had a name.

In the remnant republic named Yugoslavia, an outbreak in late 1995 and 1996 caused more than 2000 cases of HFRS, the vast majority of them a severe form. The same outbreak was seen in Croatia, a neighboring fragment of the old Yugoslavia. Across the new border in Bosnia, where a bloody war was raging, the same outbreak produced 300 victims in the Tuzla region, most of them soldiers. In a grim echo of the Korean experience, those struck down by the new disease included members of the United Nations forces stationed there. It was not the first time troops had fallen victim to such a disease there. Several thousand German soldiers had developed HFRS in Yugoslavia during World War II.

As before, the risk factors were exposure to rodents, a rural location, and agricultural activities. All were linked to disease. Again, cats seemed to be a villain rather than a savior.

Studying blood from the patients showed that Puumala, Dobrava, and possibly even Hantaan were circulating in the area, and a high proportion of the infections were caused by the new virus, with far more severe effects than those expected in European hantavirus disease. In Greece, where it was first seen, Dobrava seems to be the main cause of HFRS.

The range of the main host of Dobrava includes much of Europe, and the virus also circulates farther north, with at least one probable case in Germany and others in Belgium. The severe nature of Dobrava HFRS makes it unlikely that it has remained unnoticed in these areas in large numbers. What is clear is that there are almost certainly new hantaviruses causing human disease as yet undetected in many areas.

OTHER HANTAVIRUSES: MOSTLY HARMLESS

Any discussion of the diseases caused by hantaviruses gives only half of the picture. Hantaviruses have been identified as the causes of disease, as happened with Hantaan, Seoul, Puumala, and Dobrava, but what if there is no disease to find?

Once laboratory tests for hantaviruses were available, surveys could be carried out on rodents in many areas. One such area was the upper reaches of the Volga River in northern (European) Russia, around what is now known as Bashkortostan. The area had long been the center of what was called Tula Fever. Between 1930 and 1934, 915 cases of Tula fever had caused five deaths. In 1958 and 1959, it was recognized that this was another form of HFRS, which made this an obvious place to look for hantaviruses. Surveys of rodents in the area were reported in 1994 and identified a new hantavirus carried by the European common vole, *Microtus arvalis*. An obvious candidate to cause Tula fever, it was named Tula.

That virus, however, has still not been shown to cause any human disease. Tula fever is now known to be caused by the Puumala virus. Approximately 6000 cases of Tula fever occur annually in this region, about 25–30 times the rate of HFRS compared to other areas of Russia. Disease in children in unusually common, accounting for 493 of 9403 cases in the recent epidemic in the area. Severe infections requiring dialysis have been reported in children, although these only account for about one-third of 1% of cases. Why this region is such a focus of disease is still unknown.

Tula virus is also found in central and southern Europe as well, but has not been linked to any disease there either. So, here was a new virus but no disease. That was to happen again and again.

- Khabarovsk, in the Russian far east, carried by the reed vole, *Microtus fortis*.
- Topografov, carried by the Siberian lemming, *Lemmus sibericus*.
- Further east still, Thailand, carried by the bandicoot rat, *Bandicota indica*.
- In Japan, Tobetsu, carried by the vole *Clethrionomys rufocanus*.
- In India, Thottapalayam, carried by the musk shrew *Suncus murinus*, possibly a spillover infection from an as yet unidentified host.
- Muju virus in the main Korean vole species, *Eothenomys regulus*, sharing its space with the hantavirus that brought them all to the notice of the world.

None of them was linked to any disease in humans.

Hantavirus expert Brian Hjelle has suggested that Puumala may be the tip of the iceberg for all of the vole hantaviruses, with real but even milder diseases caused by the others. Puumala itself however, causes a disease mild enough that it usually escapes notice, so any diseases of this kind would be hard to detect. It is impossible to say unequivocally that they do not cause any disease in humans at all. If they do, they are unlikely to be major concerns.

Probably. There are no certainties, except that there are more hantaviruses out there waiting to be found.

SUBSETS OF HANTAVIRUS

Hantaviruses were falling into groups. At the genetic level, there were at least seven, but there seemed to be a more basic split. Hantaviruses are able to infect a wide range of host animals. At least 71 possible hosts were identified in one Chinese study, a number that includes *Homo sapiens sapiens:* humans. However, they all seemed to have one preferred host animal and, on that basis, they could be split:

- Those carried by voles, belonging to the rodent subfamily *Arvicolinae.* With Puumala as their most obvious member, the others seemed to cause mild or no disease.

- Those carried by the old world rats and mice of the subfamily *Murinae.* These were the bad ones. Hantaan, Seoul, and Dobrava. The killers.

- In the Americas, separated by 20 million years of evolution and two oceans, there were other rodents, the *Sigmodontinae,* different rodents with different viruses that, while hidden as yet, were killers.

LAURASIA

The story of hantaviruses in America does not begin with the recognition of hantavirus pulmonary syndrome in 1993. It does not begin with the first authenticated case in 1978 or even the first suspected case in 1959.

It begins about 20 million years ago in the early Miocene era, when the protorodents that ranged the primal supercontinent of Laurasia became separated by the parting of the land bridge between what was to become Asia and North America. The appearance of water between the two forced evolution to proceed independently on the two land masses. Rats and mice in Asia evolved into the *Murinae,* and their hantaviruses evolved with them. Those that caused human disease came to produce the kidney damage and hemorrhagic fever known as HFRS.

In the new continent of North America, a whole new subfamily of rats and mice was to evolve, the *Sigmodontinae.* As the rodents evolved, so did the viruses that lived with them.

As the land bridge between North and South America formed, about 6 million years ago at the end of the Miocene era, the rodents crossed it and established themselves in the southern half of the now united continents.

When the Beringia land bridge emerged from the lowered sea during the ice ages and humans crossed to Alaska, some time between 35,000 and 12,000 years ago, they found a whole new ecosystem.

In that ecosystem were the American hantaviruses. They did not often infect humans. When they did, they were killers beyond anything seen in Europe or Asia, but the first to be identified was apparently harmless, carried by yet another vole.

THE FIRST AMERICAN HANTAVIRUS

In 1982, Carleton Gajdusek's curiosity, one of the most prominent features of any scientist, found an unusual expression. He had a long-running interest in hantaviruses and was very curious about the lack of any native American hantaviruses. So in an example of direct action he searched the grounds of his home in Frederick, Maryland.

Working together with Ho Wang Lee, he identified a novel virus carried by a native American meadow vole, *Microtus pennsylvanicus*. The virus was named Prospect Hill, after the area where Gajdusek lived, and seemed to be most closely related to the Tula virus found in voles in European Russia.

It was widely known that the vole hantaviruses were at worst associated with mild disease. Gajdusek investigated and found that there was no human disease associated with the virus. That was to be a factor in what happened 10 years later.

AND NOT THE SECOND

In 1986, a case of fatal hemorrhage and kidney failure in a resident of Leakey, Texas, looked like hantavirus disease. When rodents were trapped, the house mouse (*Mus musculus*) was found to be carrying a hantavirus. It was named Leakey virus, and until 1992 was thought to be the second American hantavirus. When its genes were analyzed, however, it seemed to be very similar indeed to a strain of Puumala virus. This was surprising given the lack of any other identification of a Puumala-type virus in America in the intervening years. It seemed very likely that Leakey was actually a laboratory stock of Puumala virus that had somehow contaminated the tests.

Leakey virus was quietly dropped from the list.

Although it seems to be a scientific mistake, Leakey virus illustrates the processes of science rather well. It was an interesting new finding, and a new finding will be followed up. If it does not hold up, however interesting, it will be discarded. To be able to remove a theory is often as important as being able to introduce one. Given the recent finding of Muju, a new

Puumala-like virus in Korea, thousands of miles from Puumala's European home, Leakey may yet ride again.

BAD TIMING

The early 1990s were a time when federal budgets were under severe pressure. Many programs were being cut back in an effort to reduce expenditure and rein in the huge and still mounting budget deficit. Cutting was seen as good, with public opinion very much in favor of tax cuts and against government spending, except of course in programs that benefited them personally.

It is always difficult to decide what to cut back. Given the demonstrated link between rats and kidney disease in the Baltimore study, the decision to cut rodent control programs by half in that city was at least made with knowledge of the likely consequences. Around the same time, federal funding for rodent control in New York was completely removed, with large cuts in local funding as well, despite warnings from the city health commissioner that specifically mentioned her concern over rodent-borne diseases, including HFRS. Had the administrators wanted to do so, they could have pointed out the relatively limited nature of hantavirus disease in America. They could even (if they were up to date) have mentioned that scientists seemed to have decided that the hantavirus apparently carried by the house mouse was not a problem after all. At least they had some data on which to base their judgment.

Sometimes, there are no data. Sometimes a killer comes from nowhere.

RESEARCH FOR THE SOLDIER

The U.S. Army had many long-running medical research programs, working under the general rule of "research for the soldier." The United States Army Medical Research Institute of Infectious Diseases at Fort Detrick, Maryland, had a truly world-class research facility, but the real strength of any research effort is the skills and knowledge of the people who make it up. In the words of Dr. C. J. Peters, then based at USAMRIID as a colonel in charge of the Disease Assessment Division, "we at USAMRIID were caught up in the same budgetary cuts as everyone else."

As a result of these cuts, many highly skilled workers left the Army research program. Fortunately for the people of the United States and of the world, many of them did not leave the field of infectious diseases research. In fact, there seems almost to have been a pipeline for people with these specialist skills, direct to Atlanta, Georgia, and the Centers for Disease Control. C. J. Peters left USAMRIID after over 20 years to become Head of the Special Pathogens Branch in the Division of Viral and Rickettsial Diseases of the National Center for Infectious Diseases, based at the CDC. Making the same move were Drs. Jamie Childs in epidemiology and Thomas G. Ksiazek in diagnostics. They were to be major players when it became clear that hantaviruses were a very real problem for Americans within their own country, not just those a long way from home.

Among the Army research programs at that time was one at USAMRIID studying hantaviruses, with an emphasis on Asian HFRS. It was descended directly from the United Nations hospital at Uijonbu that had made such efforts to identify the cause of Korean hemorrhagic fever in the early 1950s. HFRS continued to be a problem for the Army, with a lethal outbreak among military personnel stationed in Korea as recently as 1987.

The work at USAMRIID under Drs. Connie Schmaljohn, Joel Dalrymple, and Peter Jahrling was focused on the production of viral proteins using a range of systems for use in the diagnosis of hantavirus disease and the development of possible vaccines. A vaccine for Hantaan was under development at that time and was to progress into testing for human use a few years later, and the laboratory was well established and highly productive. The staff of the laboratory at USAMRIID was to prove a vital source of the skills and techniques needed to trace hantaviruses.

It has become one of the many "accepted facts" surrounding the story of hantaviruses in the United States that the Army hantavirus research program was almost destroyed by budget cuts in 1992, a dark coincidence just months before hantavirus was found to be a deadly disease within the borders of the United States. Many sources have referred to these cuts, one stating that "budget cuts in 1991–1992 at the U.S. Department of Defense forced closure of most Army medical research programs . . . Army hantavirus research slowed radically," and also that "DOD budget cutters . . . . gutted the Army's hanta program."

However, as usual with such stories, it did not happen that way. While staff did leave USAMRIID, Dr. Schmaljohn herself says, "there was not an abolition, or even a big reduction in the amount of funding for hantavirus research in 1992, or before or after that. We have continued to receive sufficient support for all of our studies on diagnostics, vaccine development and molecular characterization of hantaviruses."

Many programs were cut, but fortunately for all concerned, the hantavirus program at USAMRIID was to remain viable and able to make a vital contribution to the coming events.

NEW VIRUSES

In working out how hantaviruses lived with their rodent hosts and their role in humans disease, scientists called on the knowledge gained with the broad range of other viruses in over 100 years of work.

In 1892, Dimitri Ivanofsky discovered that the agent of the Ukrainian tobacco disease he was investigating passed through his porcelain filters. They would stop bacteria, but not this new "filter passing virus." The discovery of viruses began there and has not stopped since: the first animal virus in 1898, the first human virus in 1901, all the way to molecular techniques that were to identify Sin Nombre in 1993 and beyond.

New techniques revealed new agents for disease, but none of them were truly new. All were 3 billion years old.

9

THREE BILLION YEARS

· · · · · · · · · · ·

I seem to have been only a boy playing on the sea-shore, and diverting myself in now and then finding a smoother pebble or a prettier shell than ordinary, whilst the great Ocean of truth lay all undiscovered before me   ISAAC NEWTON

· ·

. . . can we doubt . . . that individuals having any advantage, however slight, over others, would have the best chance of surviving and of procreating their kind?

CHARLES DARWIN, *The Origin of Species,* 1859

· ·

THE BASICS OF LIFE

To understand where viruses come from and how something so simple can produce such large effects requires an understanding of the basic machinery that is shared by all forms of life.

At its most fundamental, life exists to produce more life, to pass its genes on to future generations. We are vehicles to ensure the immortality of our genes. It is the same for a virus, a tulip, or a human and it is the genes themselves that contain the instructions to allow it to happen.

The instructions are contained in the code of life, the genetic code, which is written in just four letters: A, C, G, and T. These are the shorthand used to describe the subunits of deoxyribonucleic acid (DNA), the nucleotides. Each contains a sugar, a phosphate, and a *base:* adenine, cytosine, guanine, or thymine. Attached to the backbone of sugars and phosphates, these are the individual letters of the genetic code. It is the order of these four letters that code for every kind of life, from the smallest virus to the largest and most complicated creatures. Despite our human-centered view of the universe, the most complex are the flowering plants, which can have hundreds of times more genetic material than humans. In terms of the amount of DNA needed to code for how we are made, we are slightly above the potato and well below the tulip.

In the cells of every kind of life, the code is written in the millions-long paired strings of DNA, and it is this that passes from generation to generation, carrying the words of the code: the genes. The two strands of DNA are not exact copies of each other. Rather, they use a code of opposites, where C on one strand specifies G on the other (and, of course, G means C), while T means A (and A means T). This is controlled by the fitting together of the different-sized nucleotides inside the tight coil of the DNA double helix.

DNA is the information storehouse, but it needs another molecule to get the messages out into the cell, where they can be acted on. That molecule is another nucleic acid, ribonucleic acid, RNA.

RNA is short lived in cells and has another base, uracil (U) instead of thymine (T), with an extra oxygen atom in every sugar. RNA made from the DNA strand is not an exact copy, but is made using the code of opposites, a process referred to as *transcription.*

Most of the RNA made is used as messages to dictate the production of proteins, which do the actual work, whether as enzymes driving reactions or as the structure of the cell itself. Each protein is produced as a string of subunits. The use of repeating subunits makes the best use of limited information and is a very common theme in biology. In this case, each subunit is one of 20 related molecules known as amino acids. Each amino acid added to the growing protein is selected by the letters of the genetic code. Three letters of the nucleic acid code decide one letter of the protein code, and each RNA molecule can be used again and again to make multiple copies of its protein, a process known as *translation.* Once made, these amino acid chains form the backbone of the mature protein, which is folded and added to by the cell based on that amino acid structure.

All of this complexity is to allow the DNA at the heart of the cell to pass itself down through time, but there was a time before the first DNA. So where did all of this come from?

LIFE

At the time of the Renaissance, the blooming of science in Europe after the Middle Ages, it was widely believed that life arose spontaneously all the time. There was no understanding of the complexity of life at the biochemical level. Spoilage of food by molds was thought to be by the generation of the mold from within the food itself. Maggots were thought to be generated by the rotting of meat.

This belief was not held true for only simple forms of life. A recipe for mice was published in the 17th century: after a mixture of old shirts and wheat was placed in a jar, it took 21 days for the mixture to produce mice. The idea that mice came into the well-provisioned nest from outside was not considered.

The first real challenge to the idea that life "just appeared" came in 1668 with the demonstration by Italian physician Francesco Redi that maggots did not appear in rotting meat if flies were kept away by gauze screens. The debate continued, however.

In 1674, Antoni van Leeuwenhoek's first microscopes showed "little animalcules" in water. This appeared to support the idea of spontaneous generation of life because the animalcules would appear in "simple mixtures" such as hay in water.

In 1745, the English clergyman John Needham showed that the little animalcules would appear even in boiled broth, "proving" that life arose spontaneously. However, when another priest, Lazzaro Spallanzani, showed that if the air was evacuated and the broth was boiled in the flask rather than tipped in after boiling, life did not appear. Supporters of spontaneous generation argued that his results proved only that air was needed to create life.

Then in 1859, Louis Pasteur, at the time a professor in Strasbourg, showed that even if air was allowed into the flask, life did not appear. He used boiled meat broth in flasks with long, thin curved necks. As we now know, it was bacteria in the air entering the flask that caused life to "appear," and in Pasteur's flask they settled out in the thin curves of the glass neck. When the flask was tilted to allow the broth to wash into the neck, life "appeared." Pasteur showed that the air itself contains life, but that life does not simply appear. Rather, it all goes back billions of years to events in another broth, the "primordial soup."

A RECIPE FOR SOUP

Life as we know it today is hugely complicated at the chemical level. Yet it is thought that all of that vast complexity originated in the complex brew of unliving chemicals that is referred to as the "primordial soup." The Earth in that early time was far from what it is now: a poisonous atmosphere, swirling above dead seas, wracked by the violent storms and volcanic eruptions of the young planet, with harsh sunlight battering down.

Humans tend to think of what they see as the way things have always been, but we are seeing the end of billions of years of change. The biology of evolution is even more lacking in certainty than other areas of science because while we can travel almost anywhere on the Earth, we can only view the past through memories and records. The whole of mankind's recorded history is no more than a few thousand years, while life originated on Earth billions of years ago. There are stories in the rocks, however, for those who can read them.

In 1924, the Russian biochemist Alexandr Ivanovich Oparin proposed that the earliest forms of life appeared in the seas of the primeval earth, formed from simple molecules in reactions powered by the fierce sunlight. From studying ancient rocks, he found evidence that the early atmosphere was totally different from that of the modern world. There was no free oxygen. Instead there was methane, carbon dioxide, ammonia, nitrogen, water, and hydrogen.

All of the oxygen in the atmosphere, which we think of as essential to life, is actually thought to have come from living creatures, killing many of them as the concentration increased, until forms of life came into being that needed it rather than produced it: us.

In that primordial mixture over 3 billion years ago, life had its beginnings. Random chance produced molecules that could copy themselves.

And that is not just theory.

Laboratory experiments by Stanley Miller in 1953 used water under an atmosphere of hydrogen, methane and ammonia. Energy came from electrical discharges, simulating the lightning storms of a young earth. It took only 1 week to generate amino acids, the basic building blocks of proteins. Similar experiments since then have generated nucleotides, the building blocks of nucleic acids.

And this is on a human time scale. A billion years opens depths of possibility beyond human knowing.

FOSSILS

In life as it is today, RNA is the servant of the genes, a messenger molecule carrying instructions from the DNA out into the machinery of the cell. However, evidence shows that RNA is actually a molecular fossil of the earliest forms of life. While DNA needs proteins to unwind it, copy it, cut it and repair its almost endless chains, the smaller RNAs can do much of this for themselves. It was the discovery in 1986 of RNA molecules that could cut and join themselves that showed that RNA could have been the start of all life.

While we cannot know exactly what happened in the primordial soup, just one molecule that was able to copy itself had to appear for all life to begin.

COMPLEXITY

What those first elements of life looked like will remain forever unknowable to us unless time itself is no longer a barrier. Yet in the spectrum of life around us we see almost all levels of complexity.

This is an argument used by those who cannot believe that random events could have produced what we see around us. To creationists, there "has not been enough time" for evolution to have produced the staggering complexity we see in even the simplest life. But even around us we can see evidence for time beyond our imaginings.

The land of the Four Corners provides a convincing lesson that time extends outside human comprehension. Canyons a mile deep, cut by the tiny thread of a river, one grain of sand at a time drifting downstream to open the unimaginable depths. Even before that, tiny specks falling through a primordial sea to compress and fuse, crushed by a billion minuscule weights above them, forming the mile-thick layers we call sandstone, one grain at a time. To look on such things is to realize that the span of humans is a thin skin on the surface of creation.

We can picture the first self-replicating molecules bunching together, maybe with an outer layer of tougher molecules for protection. As time passed, time that human minds can only dimly imagine, these crude bundles began to evolve into the first cells, drawing different elements into themselves and from within themselves.

By the most basic law of evolution, those that could grow did. Those that could not compete died out. This is survival of the fittest, natural selection. It works at every stage, from the first molecule to the first human.

The subunits of the DNA that forms the genes of cells are only one atom of oxygen different from those of RNA, a simple change at the molecular level. Proteins are the machinery of the cell, but RNA makes the proteins. The key elements in the formation of protein are three different kinds of RNA that match and align the amino acids that form the protein, following instructions from the code in the genes. Even today, in viruses, sometimes those genes can be RNA.

So there is a path from the first self-copying molecules to the vast complexities that are life as we know it today.

CELLS TO CELLS

Even when cells had appeared, change continued. Our own cells are far larger and more complex than the simple cells of bacteria, which probably look more like some of the earliest cells. Bacteria are a different kind of life than that we can see around us. Bacterial cells are smaller and far simpler than the cells that make up the more complex life forms, but they allow bacteria to have a whole life cycle, growing and reproducing using simple nutrients and light or chemical energy. Without bacteria, we could not live. The parts of the cell that generate energy and the parts of plant cells that use energy of light to make the building blocks of life are all highly evolved forms of bacteria that came to live within our cells in the unimaginable past. They have their own genes, and these, together with the genes of the cell itself, pass the instructions to each new generation.

While most genes stayed within cells, using the machinery of the cells to pass themselves down through time, some genes developed the ability to go it alone.

THE MAKING OF A VIRUS

Where the first virus came from is unknown. Because a virus needs a cell to allow it to grow, viruses could not have been the first forms of life. The relics of these early living molecules may exist, but are most likely to be found within cells themselves. Rather, it seems likely that viruses arose as genes that became able to move within the cell. We still see these in the circular nucleic acids known as *plasmids,* found in bacteria and able to pass themselves into new cells. Mobile genes are found in almost every form of life where we have looked for them.

Then, by picking up a protective coat of protein and, more importantly, the genes to make that coat for every new generation, some of these genes became able to move out of the cell and look for new cells to host them. Natural selection was acting at every stage to make them more able to grow and infect, with the less efficient versions falling away with every generation. They evolved to be able to select those target cells that would allow them to grow. They evolved to alter those cells into factories to make more of this new form of life.

The first viruses.

WHAT IS A VIRUS?

However they evolved, which is still a matter that is debated hotly, a virus is simply a set of coded instructions to the right kind of cell, telling it how to make more viruses. What a virus has to do is to redirect the machinery of the cell, whatever the cell tries to do about it.

Some viruses have genetic material like that of the cell, made of DNA, and need to use much of the cellular machinery. Others, more complicated, with more DNA genes, make most of their own machinery and only need to use the basic structure of the cell. Most viruses exist in the RNA world, however, themselves living reminders of the mechanisms of that distant past. They do not, ever, make DNA.

Because RNA is shorter lived than DNA, it is not repaired in the same way as DNA and cells do not copy it with so much care. With DNA, as the copy is made, each added nucleotide is checked. If it is wrong, it is removed and the cell tries again until it gets it right. Being less important, RNA does not get this "proofreading," so the RNA used by some viruses to carry their genetic code changes a million times faster than DNA, allowing them to mutate their genes at hugely increased rates. This is key in getting around host defenses and the effects of antiviral drugs. The rate of change is so fast that it is very unlikely that any RNA virus is an exact copy of its parent.

The collection of genes, referred to as the *genome*, whether carried on RNA or on DNA, is what makes the virus. In some cases the genome alone can be used to infect cells, although of course it is far less efficient than the whole virus, which is actually a custom-designed genome transport.

Viruses using RNA to carry their genes cannot use the cellular machinery to copy RNA, as cells do not do this. They need to make proteins to allow this RNA-only life, but apart from this they still use much of the machinery of the cell. So viruses carry the nucleic acid code to reprogram the cell, turning it into a virus factory. However, most nucleic acids are delicate molecules, easily destroyed. RNA in particular is very fragile so the genes must be protected. To do this, all viruses wrap their delicate, vital code in a protein shell. Some go a step further and wrap that in a fatty sheath stolen from the host cell. So the code is protected.

That alone is not enough. Outside a cell, a virus is inert. It doesn't grow, it cannot change. It is a collection of chemicals—potential, not life. To copy itself, a virus must get inside the right kind of cell. It needs special proteins, coded from its genes, which stud the outside of the virus particle. These recognize structures on the surface of the correct kind of cell and get the virus inside. Some may also cut the virus free from sticky coatings that protect the cell or allow it to hide from the immune system with which the body tries to defend itself. All of this is purely and simply to get the virus into the cell. Outside the cell, the virus can do nothing. It drifts, inactive, just waiting to bump into the right structure on the right cell.

There are many viruses, however, and random chance gets enough into the right place for the next stage to happen.

INSIDE THE CELL

Once the virus attaches to the cell and gets inside, the battle has only just begun. Cells are in the business of survival as well and do not make all of their machinery for the purpose of making it available to any passing virus. Cells have their own defenses.

Infected cells will try to prevent infection of the body by committing suicide, breaking themselves apart using the "self-destruct button" known as *apoptosis*. They may also call in the cell-killing immune response. The human body is more than willing to sacrifice any cell that looks like it is infected. Many, many protections exist that a virus must counter before it can use its captured cell to make more virus.

The code in the virus must contain the genes to make proteins for its coat, proteins to allow it to get into the cell, proteins to steal the machinery of the cell, proteins to provide any missing functions that the cell does not have but which the virus needs (copying RNA, for example), and proteins to help the virus evade the immune system. All of these are spelled out in four letters of nucleic acid, coding for 20 letters of protein, coding for the whole of life.

It is common to think of viruses as intelligent, malicious creatures, outsmarting humans in their quest to destroy. This is wrong. Viruses have no intelligence, no malign nature. They are created by random chance with one drive: to multiply. If a million monkeys with a million typewriters can write Hamlet, then a billion viruses with a billion of the random changes called *mutations* can write influenza, Ebola, or nothing at all. Most of these random changes in the genetic code weaken the virus, making it less able to survive, but there are so many that a few, a very few, are stronger. They can dodge the immune system, evade some new drug, or maybe just grow that little bit faster. These few make the next generation. What happens to the rest does not matter to the virus.

HOW DO VIRUSES SPREAD?

The next generation of viruses has to spread. Early in the infection of an individual host, this probably just involves finding another cell close by. At some point, however, the virus needs to spread to a new host. There are a range of routes it can use, which have a huge effect on the efficiency with which it spreads.

Viruses that cause large epidemics tend to spread efficiently, and one of the most efficient routes of all is by air: aerosol spread. Some viruses infect the lungs or the tubes leading to the lungs and convert the cells lining the passages into virus factories. Huge quantities of the virus are breathed out by the infected host. Examples of this route include influenza or any of the huge range of viruses that cause the common cold.

Other viruses get into the air by different routes. Aerosols can be generated in many ways, such as by the bursting of blisters on the skin as with measles or chickenpox. In the case of hantaviruses, the aerosol is generated as dust from nests or other material contaminated by rodent excretions. So while there is a great deal of concern about aerosol spread of "killer viruses," just using this route does not mean that they will continue to spread among humans. Hantaviruses, for example, enter humans by the aerosol route but, with few exceptions, they do not leave.

Another route that can be an efficient means of spreading a virus is the fecal–oral route. This relies on contamination of food or (most often) drinking water with sewage. A related route is by excretion in the urine, using the same method of entry. These routes are very important in the spread of diarrhea viruses and even some types of hepatitis. Clearly this is less of a problem in wealthier societies, where clean drinking water is commonly available, but it is a major route of infection in crowded urban slums and also in certain rural settings. Many diseases of animal origin can also infect humans by this route, and there are cases where hantaviruses appear to have been transmitted directly in rodent urine.

Spread by aerosol or by the fecal–oral route can allow one individual to infect a huge number of others rapidly and effectively. A less rapid route of spread is by body fluids. This can be very efficient, as the AIDS epidemic clearly demonstrates, but is slower, allowing only a limited number of people to be infected by one individual. Viruses spread by this route are often spread by sexual contact or by the use of contaminated needles, either for drug abuse or by the reuse of needles in poorly equipped hospitals. Ebola is spread by this route, and it is often nursing care of the infected victim that spreads that particular killer.

Sometimes a helper is used to spread the virus. Most often, this is a biting insect or mite. Again, this can be a very efficient method of spread, allowing one host to spread the infection to many others. Yellow fever, Rift Valley fever, and other, nonviral, infections such as malaria are spread by this route. Rift Valley fever is a cousin to the hantaviruses and is described in more detail later on.

WHERE DO VIRUSES COME FROM?

What we now know to be Hantaan hantavirus disease was first reported in 960 A.D., but the virus causing it was not identified for a thousand years. Even with hantavirus pulmonary syndrome, where the disease itself was newly identified, the virus had been living with its host mouse for thousands, maybe even millions of years, and had been causing human disease for much of that time.

Just because humans do not know something exists does not make it new when it is finally discovered. As the "New" World had formed 6 million years before the arrival of mankind over the Beringia land bridge or across the Atlantic, so many "new" viruses are more accurately described as "unknown."

Of course, viruses are evolving all the time, but the time scale involved is too slow for us to see it happening. The slow drift of random mutation is constantly changing every biological organism, but a human lifetime is just not long enough to see it.

Viruses can appear through any of a bewildering variety of routes. Many paths exist for a virus to enter a human population. Indeed, at the most basic level, any change can expose humans to new diseases.

NEW VIRUSES

There is no such thing as new life. There hasn't been for billions of years. All that exists is life that has evolved from some other form of life.

As there is no new life, so there are no new viruses. Yes, viruses can appear where they have not been seen before. They can change, allowing them to infect a new host. They can alter their structure so that they are not recognized by the defensive mechanisms of the body or they can simply be discovered, but they are not "new." Not unless shirts and wheat really do make mice.

10

ON THE ORIGIN OF VIRUSES
· ·

It is interesting to contemplate an entangled bank, clothed with many plants of many kinds, with birds singing on the bushes, with various insects flitting about, and with worms crawling through the damp earth, and to reflect that these elaborately constructed forms, so different from each other, and dependent upon each other in so complex a manner, have all been produced by laws acting around us.

CHARLES DARWIN, *The Origin of Species,* 1859
· ·

EMERGING VIRUSES

Viruses perceived as "new" are not necessarily even changed; most are more accurately described as "emerging," defined by the Centers for Disease Control as: "A disease of infectious origin with an incidence that has increased within the last two decades, or threatens to increase in the near future."

Many diseases fit this definition, but most publicity has focused on the viruses that cause incurable, fatal diseases such as Ebola, hantavirus pulmonary syndrome, or the acquired immune deficiency syndrome, AIDS.

In general, the term "emerging disease" is most commonly applied to diseases that historically have been rarely seen (or identified). It is easier to see a change in a disease that has been restricted to a small area or has infected only small numbers of people. Indeed, even a major increase in an already common infection may be thought of as an epidemic or the worldwide epidemic known as a "pandemic" rather than an emerging disease.

Despite the entirely justified attention given to lethal diseases, many less spectacular diseases also fit the CDC definition. In fact, it is not even necessary for an emerging disease to be caused by a rare or novel virus. In countries where the vaccine is not yet available, chicken pox in adults is increasing. This is traditionally an uncommon disease outside the tropics, but it is becoming far more common as infection with the virus during childhood has been prevented by anxious parents. Unfortunately, adult chicken pox is far more severe, often causing serious lung infections, and the increase in the disease is a cause for concern. Despite the emerging nature of the disease, the virus itself is neither novel nor rare.

It is clear that even the emergence of infections is not new. It has happened throughout history and covers the whole range of infections, from the trivial (and often unnoticed) up to the high-profile killers.

WHY DO VIRUSES KILL?

Viruses do not need to kill their host to grow. In fact, many do not cause any apparent harm to the host. They grow in a few cells, maybe not even killing those cells, and they wait. When a virus does kill, that is often a sign that it is poorly adapted to a host. Viruses that have had time to adapt to their host often cause only mild or unnoticeable disease. Often, but not always.

The classical theory states that it is in the interest of a virus not to kill or immobilize the host too quickly, as this reduces the chances for spread of the virus. Over time, both virus and host adapt so that the virus produces less severe disease in its normal host. The best example of this is myxomatosis in the Australian rabbit population.

In a strikingly ill-advised attempt to provide a useful source of meat and fur, a limited population of European rabbits was introduced to Australia in the 19th century. They escaped and multiplied rapidly. By the 20th century they were a massively destructive and costly pest, and no control method worked. So, biological warfare was used.

Myxoma virus is related to human smallpox, but causes an infection only in rabbits. In American rabbits (the normal host) this virus causes mild and self-limiting skin disease. Despite their outward similarity, European rabbits are a different species. They are different enough that in them the virus causes myxomatosis, a severe systemic disease lethal to more than 90% of infected rabbits. The virus was released into the Australian rabbit population of the Murray River valley in 1950 in an attempt to control their numbers. It was transmitted very efficiently by the huge numbers of mosquitoes that prey on the rabbits. In the short term it was highly effective, wiping out over 99% of the rabbits across a huge area of Australia.

Within 7 years, though, three quarters of the rabbits survived infection due to natural selection of disease-resistant rabbits combined with the evolution of less lethal viruses that allowed their hosts to survive longer. The advantage of disease resistance to the rabbit is obvious, but why did the virus adapt to become less lethal?

In winter, rabbits retreat into their burrows and come into far less contact with other rabbits. The number of mosquitoes is far lower, and a rapidly lethal virus that infects a rabbit at the start of winter will kill the rabbit in its burrow before the virus has a chance to spread. If the virus has changed to cause a milder infection, so that the rabbit is still alive in the spring, the new crop of mosquitoes can spread the virus to new hosts. So, less lethal viruses are spread more effectively.

As a result of this selection of both rabbit and virus, a general immunity to the virus became established so that by 1960 the rabbit population was recovering rapidly, even though the virus was still present and circulating among them.

As with myxomatosis in the early stages of the Australian epidemic, when a novel host is infected, there has been no chance for adaptation to a less virulent form, and severe disease may result. The newly introduced virus was a horribly efficient killer, but once both host and virus had adapted, the two could coexist.

A more extreme form of the benign adaptation hypothesis has also been suggested. Symbiosis is a coexistence of two species, from which both gain an advantage. Under the theory of "aggressive symbiosis," often referred to as the "virus X" theory after the book in which it was proposed, viruses may act to benefit their host by providing a defense against "invaders." Under such a theory, fully adapted viruses could, while not harming their natural host, infect a new species with which the host comes into contact, helping the normal host to win out in competition with the sickened opponent species.

The theory fits well with the many primate viruses that can infect and cause severe disease in the closely related human species. We are, after all, just an overachieving plains ape in evolutionary terms.

However, there are problems with the theory.

First, many viruses are still highly virulent in, and specific to, the normal host, and it is difficult to see the evolutionary advantage of a virus such as smallpox, which only infected humans but killed millions upon millions of people.

Second, many viruses do not cause disease, even though they can jump between species. A good example of this is one form of the usually deadly Ebola, the Reston strain described in "The Hot Zone." Most strains of Ebola are appallingly efficient killers of humans, with the death rate from Ebola Zaire infection standing at up to 90%. Ebola Reston was a fatal disease for monkeys and was able to transfer to humans, but it did not cause any human disease. Many hantaviruses fit this description as well.

Third, it is difficult to see the evolutionary advantage to the host species of some such diseases, for example, the lethal infection of humans by other hantaviruses. It's egocentric to believe humans have much influence over the world inhabited by desert mice.

Viruses clearly do coadapt with their host to reduce virulence, and new hosts often suffer from severe effects of infection. As with all simple theories, however, this one cannot hold up for every case in complex biological systems. As always, it is an intricate mix of factors that produces the final result.

Sometimes a virus does not need to jump species to be a new and deadly killer.

THE ARRIVAL OF VIRUSES

In the predominantly agricultural society with little travel between regions that has existed for most of recorded human history, it has been possible for viruses to exist in isolated areas of infection. However, as society develops, trade routes are established that allow for the transmission of infections between such areas. As more and more people travel, such transmission becomes more common along the trade routes. Military expeditions can also be responsible for spreading infection. The Spanish conquistadores under Hernán Cortés conquered the powerful Aztec nation with what looks like ridiculous ease. Why? There are many theories. Was it that a messenger from the East was seen as a spirit of the snake god Quetzalcoatl? Was it the Spaniards' use of gunpowder or horses? Was it due more to European viral infections (including smallpox and measles) passed to the totally nonimmune native population? As usual, it was a combination of factors acting together to produce the final result. However, it cannot be disputed that when the conquistadores reached some Aztec towns, they found them almost totally empty, the population having died from the new diseases or fled in terror from them. Seeing the European soldiers (who had a long history of exposure to these viruses and so were mostly immune) apparently marching unhurt through a cloud of pestilence only added to the terror.

Sometimes, like myxomatosis, the arrival of smallpox was no accident, as with the blankets Colonel Henry Bouquet arranged to provide to his Indian foes.

MAKING THE JUMP

What is clear is that a virus jumping to a new host can cause unusually severe disease; it is one of the main ways that new infections appear. When infections jump from an animal to a human they are called "zoonoses," and many of the most severe diseases of humans fall into this category.

Why jump? The key here, as always, is evolution. What can be a disadvantage under some conditions can become a significant advantage under others. Consider the following: If a virus is circulating in a large, stable population of animals in an isolated setting, there is neither the need nor the opportunity to jump to another species. Even if another possible host is present, any virus that mutates and gains the ability to jump will almost certainly reduce its ability to circulate in its normal host and so lose out because virus still circulating in the normal host will grow faster. This is not to say that it does not happen; just that the advantage is less, so it happens less often.

What if that normal host is under pressure, perhaps from the destruction of its environment by slash and burn agriculture, new construction, or ranching? Individual hosts will be stressed and be more likely to show disease. Because there will be fewer of them around, the virus cannot circulate as well. Instead of being a disadvantage, being able to make the jump to a new host can now be a real advantage. Those few viruses that have that ability are now favored, so it is these viruses that can infect and grow. These viruses get to make the next generation. This is evolution in action.

It is also a two-edged sword. If humans move into an area, the changes they make may stress some species but benefit others. Even those species that benefit can cause problems. If land is cleared for growing and storing crops, the number of rodents can increase enormously. In Korea, it is rodents living around rice fields that expose workers to the deadly Hantaan virus infection. There may be less benefit to the virus in jumping to humans, but in this setting there is enough exposure to allow any potential problem to develop to its full extent.

ATTRACTING ATTENTION

For a virus to be noticed without detailed investigations, it must cause disease in humans. In its original host, to which it has adapted, a potentially zoonotic virus may be able to circulate without drawing attention to itself. When the virus jumps to humans, to which it is not adapted, it can behave differently. Although in most cases it will not cause any significant disease, in a few cases it will, and in these cases, the lack of adaptation to the host can cause far more severe disease.

Hantavirus pulmonary syndrome provides one of the best examples of this. The virus is harmless, maybe even beneficial, in the normal rodent host, but when it manages to infect a human, it kills in days. Additionally, it is not transmitted between humans; every infection has to come directly from the infected rodent. This is a classic zoonosis.

A NEW HOST

Of course, a true zoonosis is poorly transmissible between humans, as otherwise human-to-human transmission comes to dominate the spread of the virus. When this happens, it is one of the few ways that we can see a virus that is genuinely "new" to its host appearing within a short time.

A possible example of this is the human immunodeficiency virus, which seems likely to have originated as a zoonosis. HIV is similar to a virus seen in African monkeys, the simian immunodeficiency virus (SIV). Transmission from an African ape to humans seems to be the most probable route, and has been suggested by some sources to have occurred by improbable, impractical, and highly insulting routes. These are not necessary. When skinning an ape caught for food with a blunt knife, it is highly likely that blood will mix. That is all that is required.

Even if HIV infection was originally a zoonosis, it is now a transmissible disease within the human population, and infection is by spread between humans rather than by zoonosis. Here is one virus that has found a much more promising niche in the environment than a small and endangered population of African monkeys. It has infected 30 million humans. There are 5 billion more, spread worldwide, and the virus is using its new niche to full effect.

A HELPING BITE

Although, as with HPS, an infection may spread directly from a mammalian species to humans, the transfer of many infections involves carriage by another "vector" species, which is often an *arthropod*. The name means "jointed legs" and covers a huge class of creatures, including insect, spiders, mites, and ticks. The virus is acquired when the vector feeds on the blood of the host. While it is possible for the virus to be transferred passively if a new host is bitten soon afterward, more commonly the virus grows in the arthropod vector. In some cases, the virus may even be passed to subsequent generations of the vector in the eggs.

A functional classification of such diseases as arthropod-borne viruses (arboviruses) has been widely used. It is not a formal virus name, but is still a useful designation. There are well over a hundred arbovirus infections of humans, including yellow fever, Dengue fever, and many others.

This category includes even close relatives of the hantaviruses. A cousin to hantaviruses, Rift Valley fever is in the same family of viruses, the Bunyaviridae.

OUT OF THE RIFT

Rift Valley fever is worth considering in some detail. Although it is closely related to the hantaviruses, it is a very different disease with very different mechanisms of spread. However, some of the events seen with Rift Valley fever show what could happen to its cousins.

Rift Valley fever is a disease seen in epidemics of domesticated animals (cattle, goats, and sheep) in Africa, and it kills with horrifying efficiency. During December 1997, one Kenyan family lost all but 4 of their 200 goats within 1 month. In Egypt in 1977–1978, it destroyed almost the entire meat herd of sheep, cattle, and goats across the whole country.

Sometimes it spreads to humans, either by mosquito bite or direct from the animal. When it does, it causes a severe flu-like illness in most, with eye problems caused by small hemorrhages within the eye in about 1 in 10. In one or two out of every hundred, however, the hemorrhages do not occur in the eye; they occur throughout the body.

This is called hemorrhagic fever, and it is the way that so many of the most deadly viruses kill. Within the body, the blood vessels themselves are attacked, and hemorrhages appear scattered throughout the organs. Bleeding into the body is uncontrolled.

With Rift Valley fever, there is headache, sometimes the lethal swelling of the brain known as encephalitis, pain, fever, bloody diarrhea, and bloody vomit. Then, toward the end, blood flows from the mouth and nose. Within a day, death results. Of the patients who develop Rift Valley hemorrhagic fever, more than half will die.

Rift Valley fever does not cause small outbreaks. The first to come to the attention of Western medicine was in Egypt in 1977–1978, when 200,000 people were infected and almost 600 died. In Kenya and Somalia in 1997–1998, 90,000 people were infected and 300 died.

The virus lives in mosquitoes of the *Aedes* type, and between outbreaks it is passed down to the next generation in their eggs. Most viruses of this type have what is called a *sylvatic cycle,* where they are maintained between outbreaks by transfer between wild animals, with mosquitoes acting to transfer the disease from the sylvatic host into humans or domestic animals. In in the case of Rift Valley fever, the virus seems to be so well adapted to its life in the mosquitoes that it does not need a sylvatic cycle.

These mosquitoes are normally present at low levels, but when heavy rains come to east Africa, the flooded pools known as *dambos* provide perfect breeding grounds. In 1997 the El Niño surface temperature changes in the Pacific Ocean brought drenching rainstorms to eastern Africa, flooding huge areas. Many villages were inaccessible, and the inhabitants were exposed to huge numbers of mosquitoes, with only diseased animals to eat. Some ate them and died. Even if they did not, the mosquitoes were biting.

What can be done? In the words of the Centers for Disease Control: "No vaccine for human use is available. No effective antiviral medication is approved for use in humans."

There has been preliminary work. Trials in mice and monkeys showed that the antiviral drug ribavirin could moderate the disease even when given well after symptoms developed. Ribavirin is expensive and very ineffective when given by mouth. It has to be given directly into the blood, and the clean needles to allow this to be done safely are not available in rural Africa.

A vaccine was developed more than 20 years ago, but it is still experimental. Again, it costs too much to be useful on any large scale where the disease is killing people. So, as yet, this killer is free to carry on doing what it does best.

BIOWAR

It was noted in 1977 that the Egyptian Rift Valley fever virus had some strange properties. It was far more lethal to rats and to cells grown in the laboratory than other samples of the virus. This led to rumors that it was a biological weapon, developed by the Egyptians, the Russians, the Israelis, or some other entity. No evidence for that has ever been found, but it is very common that any outbreak of disease is blamed on "them." It is a basic human need to blame someone for bad events, and infectious diseases are no different.

Sometimes the fears are true. Modern treaties prohibiting biological warfare have proven unsuccessful in preventing the development of such weapons, and only states sign treaties. Terrorists have proven repeatedly that they can obtain biological weapons. It is not only their use that presents dangers to the human populace, their very existence is a risk because containment is not guaranteed.

In 1978, in Sverdlovsk, Soviet Russia, there was an outbreak of the virulent bacterial disease anthrax. This in itself was not that unusual. There have been outbreaks before and since in Russia, usually associated with working with wool, horsehair, or other animal products. However, it was known even then that the Soviet biological warfare effort was developing antibiotic-resistant anthrax for battlefield use. Anthrax spores are stable, spread easily by dispersal in the air, and cause a lung infection (pulmonary anthrax) that can choke the victim to death within hours. It is an ideal weapon, and interest in weaponized anthrax is still very much in the news, both as a potential terrorist weapon within the United States and in Saddam Hussein's arsenal in Iraq.

Why was the Sverdlovsk outbreak suspicious? Very unusually, it involved multiple strains of bacteria. This is not seen in natural outbreaks where the infection comes from one source. In 1992, Russian President Boris Yeltsin said in the case of the Sverdlovsk outbreak, "The KGB admitted that our military developments were the cause." It has still not been admitted what these developments were at Sverdlovsk, but in this case the suspicions were correct.

Claims of production as biological warfare agents have been made for many other viruses. In the case of the human immunodeficiency virus, these were even published in the mainstream British press. Sadly for the conspiracy theorists, HIV appeared long before the technology to assemble a virus was available. To this day, nobody has the ability to make a virus as subtle, deadly, and flexible as HIV.

The suspicion also touched hantavirus. The headline "Were Four Corners Victims Biowar Casualties?" appeared in the November 1993 edition of the highly respected periodical *Scientific American.*

The short answer is "no," but the article was a measured summary of the fears expressed in the area in response to this shocking new disease. We now know that this particular hantavirus has been around for a very long time, but in the initial panic of the outbreak, the need to assign blame was strong.

In the case of Rift Valley fever, the virus appears to have changed itself without help from humans. It was clear that the 1977 Egyptian strain of Rift Valley fever did seem to be a new, more deadly version of the virus. No one knows why. It could have been mutation or an exchange of genes with a related virus. Whatever caused the change, it was different, and what can happen to one hantavirus could happen to another.

MAKING THE CHANGE

What are the current limits of genetic engineering? Can we really make a new virus?

Probably not, but we can combine elements from viruses that already exist and leaven the mixture with genes from almost any other form of life. With the routine use of recombinant DNA technology, popularly known as genetic engineering, it is now theoretically possible to produce a virus that expresses almost any desired gene, which can be done for any of a range of reasons.

Such viruses are often used to carry genes from one host to another or to make large amounts of proteins. These viruses will only be used in the laboratory, with safeguards to prevent their escape, but some of these viruses are designed for widespread use.

TRUST ME, I'M A DOCTOR

"Viruses will only be used in the laboratory, with safeguards to prevent their escape." True. But the safeguards do not always work.

The best example of this is provided once again by Australian efforts to control the rampant European rabbit population in their country. Rabbit hemorrhagic disease is caused by a member of the family *Caliciviridae*. It was first reported in China in 1984 and spread across Europe and Asia, killing up to 95% of the rabbit population. In 1995, evaluation of the virus for the biological control of rabbits in Australia began on Wardang Island, South Australia.

"Biological control" is what biological warfare is called when humans are not the target. The testing was to address very real concerns that native Australian animals could be vulnerable to the virus. It was being tested in an isolated setting before any release. Nobody knows how, but by early 1996 the virus escaped to the Australian mainland, where it caused a devastating epidemic in the rabbit population. Although the virus was licensed as a biological control agent in Australia later that year and is now in use, the escape of the virus does illustrate the hazards of experiments.

It is estimated that 20 million rabbits died within 3 months of the release of this virus. By a twist of fate, while it does seem that disease in native species was not a problem, these species are still suffering. A lot of rabbits feed many predators. Fewer rabbits means hungry predators looking for alternative food supplies and finding them among the native animals. The Australian experience also proves that no matter how noble our intentions may be, humans cannot simply pluck one link from the food chain without rattling its entire length.

Escape from the laboratory has also happened with human killers. The elimination of smallpox is the greatest success story of mankind's struggle against viruses and a powerful demonstration of the effectiveness of vaccines. The symptoms of the disease are hideous, and the virus has killed tens of millions of humans. Following an eradication campaign begun in 1958, the last "wild" case of the more severe variola major form of smallpox occurred in Bangladesh in 1975, and the last case of the milder variola minor form occurred in Somalia in 1977. It was decreed that a period of 10 years was required before smallpox could be declared eradicated.

In 1979 two cases of smallpox occurred (with one death) following a laboratory accident at the University of Birmingham, England. The outbreak was contained to just these two cases, but the release of this "extinct" virus was to bring about one more death: the suicide of the head of the laboratory concerned.

Despite this, smallpox is now officially eradicated. The last remaining stocks of the virus (held in Novosibirsk, Russia, and at the Centers for Disease Control in Atlanta) are now scheduled to be destroyed on June 30, 1999, at least in part because of the events in Birmingham.

While it is necessary to work with deadly viruses to know how to avoid their effects, the safeguards needed must be tight. Many organizations, codes, rules, and regulations exist purely to ensure this. These apply to genetically engineered viruses as well. However, some viruses are intended to get out of the laboratory.

WAR WITH THE INSECTS

Baculoviruses are viruses of insects and are widely used to express genes from other sources. Many baculoviruses produce massive amounts of a specialized protein to form a protective capsule around the virus. The mechanisms that drive the overproduction of this protein are harnessed in the laboratory, but baculoviruses exist in the wild as well, where they cause highly species-specific and virulent disease in a wide range of insect species. The protective capsule makes the virus very stable, until it is eaten by a caterpillar, when the capsule breaks down and releases the virus into its gut, starting off a lethal infection.

This combination of stability and lethality to destructive insect pests meant that baculoviruses were in themselves promising biological insecticides. Multiple baculovirus preparations for the control of a wide range of crop-destroying insects are on sale. Although they can be highly effective insecticides, they tend to be slower acting than chemical insecticides. A farmer whose crops are being eaten wants the pest dead—now. As a result, baculoviruses have been developed that are more rapidly lethal to their insect hosts. Such genes include proteins that interfere with insect chemistry as well as with insect-specific toxins. In some cases the effect of these toxins is similar to that of chemical insecticides, with the major advantage that they are produced within (and only within) the insect itself. Extensive testing and trials are being undertaken, and it is very unlikely that any such virus will threaten humans, but for the insect target they will represent a significant new disease. This too is biological warfare.

FRIENDLY VIRUSES

Some genetically engineered viruses are being prepared for human use. If these carry extra genes, these of course will be for "good" proteins rather than toxic ones. In a vaccine, the virus will be a weakened form of a virus, usually one already used as a vaccine. It may be just that, with genes removed to make it less able to cause disease. If it has extra genes, these will be chosen to target the immune system against another disease. One that is already in use is a version of the vaccinia poxvirus that was used to eliminate the closely related smallpox virus.

The engineered version of this contains a gene from rabies virus spliced into a weakened form of the vaccinia virus. The vaccine is used for preventing rabies in wild animal populations, particularly foxes. It is given inside an edible capsule and is thought to enter the bloodstream of the fox by way of cuts inside the mouth. The recombinant vaccine has been in used in the field since 1987 with no significant health concerns and appears to be effective in controlling rabies in wild fox and racoon populations.

For the new technique of "gene therapy," the engineered viruses will be selected and designed to infect the correct kind of cell within the body, carrying a "correct" version of a gene that is faulty in the intended recipient. As of yet, however, no such viruses have been released for general use.

It is important to remember that none of these techniques is new. Nature herself has been making changes for as long as there has been life on this planet.

11

CHANGES, CONCEALMENT, AND TROJAN HORSES

The chessboard is the world, the pieces are the phenomena of the universe, the rules of the game are what we call the laws of Nature. The player on the other side of the board is hidden from us. THOMAS HUXLEY, *A Liberal Education,* 1868

LITTLE CHANGES

How do "natural" changes to the genes happen? The most common route is by random change: mutation.

Evolution is driven by the slow tick of mutation. It proceeds faster for RNA than DNA and faster for viruses than for cells, as viruses produce such huge numbers of each new generation that changes are more likely. All viruses must at some time have arisen by mutation, but it is usually a slow process. Most mutations are the change of one letter of the genetic code, known as "point mutations." Sometimes bigger changes happen, with the loss or addition of a region of the nucleic acid. Many changes have no apparent effect.

That is not always true, however. Sometimes even a tiny change can have huge effects. There we can look to influenza, not in humans, but in chickens.

Influenza is a disease not just of humans but of many other species. There are three basic types of influenza, named A, B, and C. Influenza A causes the worldwide infections known as pandemics.

Each virus is a twisted core of protein containing the RNA coding for the virus genes, surrounded by a fatty sheath studded with viral proteins. These surface proteins (or antigens) of influenza virus are used to identify strains within the major types. There are two of these surface proteins: hemagglutinin (HA, which sticks to cells and is the main target of the immune system) and neuraminidase (NA, which releases the virus if it attaches where it cannot infect). These proteins are used to type the virus by testing them against antibodies raised against known types. The virus is then classified by which types of these proteins are on its surface.

Many of the known varieties of influenza actually circulate in birds. In April 1983, in a chicken house in Pennsylvania, a mild form of influenza was seen. This was not an unusual event, and the influenza was typed as H5N2. By that October, however, the virus changed dramatically. Every infected bird died.

What had happened? Surely such a huge change in the result of infection must reflect a similarly huge change in the genes of the virus?

Not this time.

A single change of one letter of the genetic code changed one letter of the three that code for an amino acid, and the amino acid lysine was inserted instead of threonine. It was a small change, but that threonine was used to attach a large and complex chain of sugars, and the new protein lacked these. These particular sugars had blocked access to a part of the protein that must be cut by specific enzymes to make the virus infectious. With the cut site open, the virus became lethal.

A small change. A big effect.

Not all changes produce any effect at all, and when they do, most are bad for the virus. Many will result in the loss of a protein that the virus needs. Others will make the virus grow less well. There are so many viruses in each generation that those very few that are changed to be more effective *will* be generated and can then outbreed all of the others. So change happens: slowly, at the level of the genes, but with unpredictable effects, from death for the virus to death for the host.

MOVING TARGETS

This slow change has other important effects. It underlies the evolution of the virus to escape the effects of the immune system or antiviral drugs. In the case of human influenza, the effects of progressive mutations are known as *antigenic drift* and are the reason why the virus changes from year to year. It is this drift that requires a worldwide network of specialist laboratories to monitor these changes and to keep the vaccines effective from year to year.

It is also mutation that drives the appearance of drug-resistant viruses. In some ways, drug resistance in viruses is less striking than it is in bacteria. "Superbugs" that antibiotics have failed against fill the newspapers: multidrug-resistant *Staphylococcus aureus* (MRSA), tuberculosis (TB), and *Streptococcus*. All are new versions of old bacterial enemies that we thought we had defeated, but by changing and exchanging genes they have countered our most deadly chemical tricks, which is why they are newsworthy. We thought we had defeated them. Antibiotics were the final answer, or so we thought.

With viruses, antiviral drugs are so new that nobody really believed that they were the "cure-all" that antibiotics seemed to be for some 50 years. With HIV, the appearance of resistance is so fast that no single drug can ever be used without the need to plan for the time when a virus will appear against which the drug will be ineffective. This is why companies around the world need to keep developing new drugs. Small changes have world-wide effects.

While escape from the effects of the immune system or drug resistance arise by mutation, this does not have to occur after a drug is used or the immune system attacks the virus. Even in any one host, mutation during normal virus growth results in the presence of a range of viruses with differing genes and differing characteristics rather than a single type. Some of these will be drug-resistant mutants. These will have changes that may be a disadvantage normally, but will be preferred when the antiviral drug to which they are resistant is used. In the same way, some will have changes that bypass the best efforts of the immune system as these develop.

These multiple types of virus present at any time are referred to as "quasi-species." They arise by mutation and mean that for almost anything we can throw at it, the virus will have an answer waiting.

There are ways around this: the simultaneous use of multiple drugs, for example, or the generation of a very broad and strong immune response. Viruses continue to use the slow step of mutation to move away from anything that might prevent them from growing, and we continue to play catch-up.

It is not always a slow dance.

SHIFT AS WELL AS DRIFT

Any virus can swap out some of its genes with a related virus or even with the genes of the cell. However, viruses do not have a system like the *plasmids* of bacteria: independent DNA circles that can hop between cells, carrying genes with them when they go. For most viruses, gene swapping requires a cut-and-join process mediated by proteins of the cell, which, while it can occur, is not common.

Some viruses have a way to get around this. Instead of having one RNA or DNA molecule containing all of the virus genes, they have several and can exchange these with any closely related virus that happens to infect the same cell. There are many viruses with this multipart, or *segmented,* genome, including many threatening to human health. For influenza A, with its eight segments, this genetic mixing can have dramatic effects.

While influenza virus surface proteins do change slowly by mutating, it is the more sudden and dramatic changes of influenza A that cause the devastating pandemics, with the same type of virus causing many millions of cases of influenza all around the world.

Influenza pandemics occur at intervals of approximately 10 to 40 years, when a type of the virus appears with completely new surface proteins to which no one is immune. When such a virus infects, a new immune response is needed, and it will be both weaker and slower than a response where the immune system has seen the virus before. Although influenza does not kill most healthy people, the lack of any immune memory of the virus allows it to cause disease.

Following disease, influenza virus is removed from the body by the immune response so that it must either spread to a new host or die. The ability to spread is vital to the influenza virus because it cannot (unlike some viruses) linger in the same host for many years.

The way in which the virus changes the proteins that mark it for destruction by the immune system is by exchanging genetic material with viruses circulating in other hosts. In the case of influenza it is thought that influenza virus from birds mixes with that from humans when both infect pigs. Recent work has clearly shown that pigs have special features that allow them to be infected by influenza viruses from both sources. Birds, humans, and pigs are brought close together by mixed farming, particularly an agriculturally efficient system referred to as pig/duck agriculture common in many areas of the developing world such as rural China. When there are few available resources, it is important to maximize efficiency, and this system allows recycling and use of wastes to produce edible meat. The influenza virus is spread very efficiently by airborne droplets, allowing it to move between animal and human with ease.

Swapping of genes is almost inevitable when two different viruses with segmented genomes infect the same host and the same cells. Most of the remixed viruses will be less able to infect, but a few may be more infectious and a very few may have the potential to cause a pandemic.

In this century, there have been three pandemic types of the surface protein known as hemagglutinin (H) and two of the surface protein neuraminidase (N). The most recent pandemics were of H3N2 influenza virus (Hong Kong flu of 1968) and H1N1 influenza virus (Russian flu of 1977, which despite the name came from the Anshan Province in northern China).

While the surface proteins can change slightly by mutating, this does not produce totally new hemagglutinin or neuraminidase , so immunity to the old type is at least partially protective. However, a sudden change to a totally new type by the genetic mixing called *antigenic shift* (as opposed to antigenic drift) produces the totally new viruses that can cause pandemics.

The worst recorded pandemic was the "Spanish" flu of 1918–1920, caused by a virus typed as Hsw1N1, since the hemagglutinin looked like one seen in pigs (swine). A new and lethal disease, it killed by a sudden massive onset of respiratory disease, flooding the lungs; this one killed worldwide. According to most estimates, this virus killed more than 20 million people. Some estimates go up to 80 million.

Following disease, the virus was cleared. The pandemic ended when enough people were immune to prevent the virus spreading to new hosts, and the virus vanished. It was typed many years later by looking at antibodies in blood samples taken at the time. Samples of the virus genes have been recovered from the remains of influenza casualties buried in permafrost in Alaska, and other efforts are under way in Spitzbergen, an island to the north of Norway. These may tell us why the virus was so deadly and help us to know if any new influenza is likely to be such a threat. This is important to know. Antigenic shift is happening all the time, but we cannot know whether the resultant virus is harmless or deadly until it is too late.

There are good reasons to fear the reappearance of Spanish flu. When a sudden and lethal pneumonia showed up in the Four Corners in 1993, that was one of the great fears. That time it was not influenza. At other times, in other places, it has been, but it has not (yet) been Spanish flu. Two cases of reaction to a potentially threatening influenza serve to show what can happen when reasonable caution is used without truly understanding what makes a virus deadly.

When an Hsw1N1 virus, apparently similar to the Spanish flu virus, was identified in January 1976 as causing influenza at the Fort Dix U.S. Army training base in New Jersey, the news caused something extremely close to panic. A huge program was begun to provide vaccine for every American, and almost 50 million people were vaccinated, at a final cost of $200 million. However, this was not the 1918 virus. Even though the outer proteins of the 1976 virus were apparently very similar, it could not infect humans in the same way, and only 13 cases were reported. So limited was its ability to infect humans that even a sergeant who gave mouth-to-mouth resuscitation to the recruit who was the only fatality did not become infected.

Clearly this was not the Spanish flu. What was the difference? The most likely explanation is that it is not only the surface proteins that can change the way the virus infects. Proteins inside the virus, which are not seen as much by the immune system, control how the virus grows when it gets inside the cell. Changes in these proteins can be very important in allowing the virus to grow in different hosts. This time around, by a random chance favoring humanity over the viruses, they had come out of the genetic mixing pot with a reduced ability to grow inside the human body.

Events surrounding the 1997 outbreak of H5N1 influenza in Hong Kong appear to be similar. As far as the human immune system was concerned, this was a new virus. The H5 surface protein had been seen in influenza viruses from birds, but had not been seen in viruses infecting humans before 1997. The virus seemed to have spread to humans from chickens, and existing immunity in humans would not be protective.

A massive and costly response was organized, with a 24-hour program to slaughter all of Hong Kong's 1.4 million chickens. Despite intensive surveillance, only 18 confirmed cases of human H5N1 influenza were observed. Six of those were fatal, showing that the virus caused severe disease when it did infect, but in January 1998, it was officially announced by the World Health Organization that "exposure to humans infected with the H5N1 influenza virus is unlikely to result in infection." Again, a virus with a threatening appearance proved unable to spread among humans. Analysis of the genes coding for the internal proteins of the virus indicated that they had originated from birds and that the virus had not picked up human genes.

With influenza, even though attention focuses on the surface proteins as the main targets of host antibodies, internal proteins can make the difference between an outbreak and a pandemic, but these can also be exchanged.

Although all viruses can swap genes, the presence of a segmented genome makes this more likely because no cutting and joining of the genome is required. There are many other viruses with multiple genome segments. These include the Reoviridae, a family of viruses containing the *rotaviruses,* which cause lethal diarrheas; the Arenaviridae, which include the deadly Lassa fever; and the Bunyaviridae, which include both Rift Valley fever and the hantaviruses.

Although picking up new genes is more rapid for viruses with segmented genomes, there are plenty of examples in other viruses. The sudden changes that can result are important in virus evolution. In particular, members of the family *Retroviridae,* which includes the AIDS virus, HIV, have highly developed mechanisms that allow them to exchange genes, both with other related viruses and with the retrovirus-related elements that form a large part of the genome of their hosts. This seems to be important in generating the huge diversity of HIV strains that are presenting such a challenge in the development of a vaccine. Not all retroviruses are deadly, however.

THE HIDDEN VIRUS

By some estimates, up to 10% of the mouse genome is actually viral in origin. Related elements have been identified in human DNA. Why is this and how did they get there?

Retroviruses are named from the Greek word *retro,* meaning backwards. This is because they reverse the normal flow of genetic information. In the cell, the DNA codes for RNA, and the RNA carries messages to the cell. In retroviruses, the genetic information is carried as RNA, as it is with most viruses. However, while those other viruses stay in the RNA world, retroviruses contain a unique enzyme, *reverse transcriptase,* that copies their RNA back into DNA. Once they have done this, as an essential part of their life cycle, they cut the cell's DNA and splice the DNA copy of their own genes into it. If the virus is growing actively, it will copy off new genome RNAs from this inserted DNA. The DNA itself remains mobile, able to cut itself free and move around within the cell's genome.

Many retroviruses seem to establish themselves in the host cell DNA and remain there, being copied with it, and passing with it into each new generation of cells. Some retroviruses seem so well adapted to this life-style that they lose the ability to come back out. Over time, more and more of the virus DNA is lost or altered, and the remaining elements of the virus genes are referred to as *endogenous* retroviruses. These range from apparently complete viruses down to a few genes. It is these that make up the virus-related sequences in the DNA of mice or humans. Because we do not know what they are doing, they have been blamed for everything from cancer to mad cow disease.

We do know that they can exchange genetic information with retroviruses infecting the cell. In a model system where mice were modified genetically to allow HIV to grow, it was found that the infecting HIV could exchange genes with the mouse retroviral elements in the cell's DNA. This caused a big scare, as the idea of AIDS picking up genes of animal origin is genuinely frightening. The retroviral elements in the mouse DNA could contain almost anything: genes to induce cancer or genes to make the new virus able to spread more efficiently or be able to resist drugs used against it. That was an experiment, and we can choose not to allow it to happen with the mouse genes, but such exposure is happening all the time with endogenous retroviruses in the cells of humans infected with HIV, again possibly contributing to the fast-moving target that is HIV.

Not all endogenous retroviruses are bad news. There do seem to be many more such elements in mammals than in birds, which led scientists to ask why. One fascinating theory is that they are necessary. While birds lay eggs, mammals give live birth. In terms of the immune system, this is a very difficult thing to do. The immune system has evolved over millions of years to fight any foreign invader: virus, bacteria, or parasite. Anything.

In the early days of modern medicine, it was known that giving blood from one person to another could be lethal. It was this that led to the development of blood typing and to the identification of the major groups, A, B, AB, and O, as well as to other group markers such as the Rhesus factor. With this knowledge, blood transfusions became possible.

What was the killer? Quite simply, it was the recognition of the proteins of the new blood as "foreign" by the immune system. Even the new blood could itself react to the proteins of the body into which it was introduced. Because it is not possible to explain to the immune system that this particular foreign material is "good," it reacted to it as a dangerous alien presence. Because the immune system has evolved to destroy tiny amounts of invaders before they could gain a foothold, the reaction to such a large amount of foreign material could be lethal.

While we can now give blood transfusions without these reactions, there are still major problems in organ transplants. Although the proteins recognized by the immune system on the donor organ are matched as closely as possible with those of the recipient, it is still necessary to give powerful drugs to damp down the immune response.

How is this relevant to endogenous retroviruses? There is one outstanding example of the immune system apparently being persuaded not to reject foreign material, and that is pregnancy. For 9 months, more or less, a pregnant woman carries within herself a fetus, half of whose marker proteins are her own. However, the other half come from the father, a foreigner to the mother's immune system. The placenta through which the fetus gains its food and eliminates its waste is in the closest possible contact with the blood and tissues of the mother.

So why does the mother's immune system not react to all these foreign proteins? Even though pregnant women are more susceptible to some infections, they do mount strong immune responses, so there must be some localized control. One fascinating suggestion is that this is mediated by the precise and very local expression of retrovirus-related elements. That would explain why mammals, which have placental, internal development of the fetus, have so many endogenous retroviruses. It is still a theory, but one with some interesting evidence to support it.

There are many examples of viruses that do not destroy, but if this theory is correct, these particular viruses would be essential for life.

THE TROJAN HORSE

Viruses infecting humans from an animal source can cause severe disease, and sometimes the virus does not have to make the jump. Sometimes mankind helps it along.

Organ transplants are life-saving procedures that are increasingly common. However, any time an organ from one person is introduced into another, it can carry with it a huge range of potential infections, and that is with a human organ transplanted into a human. By definition, that cannot introduce new viruses into the human population. What if the organ is from an animal?

Xenotransplantation is the transplanting of organs from one species into another. The application that is causing interest, and problems, is the use of organs from animals to provide a plentiful source for humans needing replacements. There are never enough human organs to go around. People, in general, prefer to keep their organs where they were put in the first place.

Even human organs have to be matched for the marker proteins recognized by the immune system in order to avoid an immune reaction that will reject the transplanted organ. Because organs from animals are very different to those from another human, the rejection is even stronger.

To get around this problem, two approaches have been identified. The first is the use of organs from apes, which are related quite closely to humans at the protein level. However, organs from apes can contain viruses able to infect human cells, and some ape viruses can kill. So interest switched to pigs, genetically modified to match human tissues more exactly. Pigs are roughly human sized and show many similarities to humans in the shape of their organs. Genetic modification can reduce the problems of rejection that come from the use of an organ from such a different source.

Recent work, however, has identified a retrovirus of pigs, which has been named *Circe*. This virus can also infect human cells. Further work has identified at least 40 other retrovirus-like elements in the genes of the pig.

The epidemiologists who study the development of infections are very concerned about the possibility of introducing zoonotic infections directly into patients. In a whole organ, there can be huge amounts of any infectious agent. Because the organ must be alive, it is not possible to disinfect it. In addition, people receiving pig organs would have to be treated with drugs to suppress the immune system to prevent rejection of the transplant. The recipients would not have a normal ability to control infection and could act as "amplifiers" for genuinely "new" viruses, allowing them to get into the human population. This is a major concern.

MIXED BLESSINGS

Even far less dramatic use of animal tissue has caused major problems. Simian virus 40 (SV40) is a small, DNA-containing virus and is a naturally occurring virus of macaque monkeys, in which the virus causes a long-term, low level *persistent* infection, localizing in the kidney. SV40 is not a virus known to spread to humans by any natural route. However in 1954 there was a major advance in preventing human disease. Jonas Salk, an American microbiologist, developed a vaccine against polio.

This was a particular concern at the time, because in 1952 the United States had seen a massive epidemic of the disease, with 57,879 cases. At a time when there were fresh public memories of school halls filled with rows of "iron lung" breathing machines keeping paralyzed polio victims alive, the vaccine was hailed as a huge triumph for American science.

Indeed it was. The vaccine was made up of polio virus grown in monkey kidney cells and then inactivated with formalin. It produced an immune response that protected the vaccine recipient from a lethal and highly contagious disease. It was widely used.

When preparing such an "inactivated" vaccine, the virus is grown, or *cultured,* in flasks of cells that are selected to permit it to grow efficiently. In the case of the polio virus, these were monkey kidney cells. Once the virus is grown and purified, the amount of formalin used to inactivate it is controlled carefully. Too little, and the virus is still alive. Too much, and the virus proteins are destroyed, unable to generate the protective immune response. Just enough must be used, carefully evaluated for the virus being inactivated.

What if the cells used to grow the virus also contained another virus? Undetected. More stable than the virus being grown. Still alive after the formalin treatment.

They did: SV40, a natural infection of monkey kidneys.

It is still not known exactly how many recipients of the inactivated polio vaccine received infectious SV40 along with their vaccine. Millions, for sure. The urgent question being asked was whether this virus could harm humans. No one knew.

Close relatives of SV40 caused cancer in some animals and, more recently, some have been linked to human cervical cancer. The virus itself is a very efficient cause of the cancer-like changes known as *transformation* in cultured cells. Once more, something very close to panic was the result.

Vaccination is now generally accepted as a good thing. Not everyone agrees, but the public perception is positive. The elimination of smallpox was due almost entirely to the well-coordinated use of a highly effective vaccine. Measles and polio are both one-time killer viruses that are targeted for elimination in the next few years by the World Health Organization.

In the 1950s, though, vaccination was still largely unproven. To have to admit that this new vaccine had inserted a cancer-causing virus into million of Americans was a full-blown nightmare for public health officials.

Fortunately, they did not have to.

Despite extensive (and expensive!) surveillance for over 40 years, no link between SV40-contaminated vaccine and human disease has ever been demonstrated. A very few cases have been found where SV40 is present in association with human disease, but no solid link has been established. We were lucky.

SV40 remains a very convincing illustration of the problems associated with introducing animal material into humans. Of course a vaccine can be purified, treated, and inactivated. None of this is possible with organs, which must be used as they are. It does seem likely that xenotransplantation will proceed, with very strict safeguards, but the risks of such procedures require a lot of thought. Organ transplant recipients would be ready-made amplifiers for any new virus.

AMPLIFICATION

Once a "new virus" has entered the human population, by whatever route, this does not make it an emerging disease. Many viruses do not cause significant disease in humans, and such viruses cannot truly be classified as emerging diseases, even if they become widespread. However, with improved diagnostic and epidemiological techniques, even previously unidentified viruses that usually cause only mild disease may become known.

Some of these viruses may be very widespread, such as human herpesvirus 6. This is one of the Herpesviridae, and like all of them it is present lifelong after the initial infection. It is present in over three quarters of people and causes the mild and transient rash of infants known as roseola infantum, one of the six "classic" rashes of childhood. It has also been linked to more severe diseases, including a very severe hepatitis. Despite this it was not identified until 1986, and the virus was only identified by isolation from an AIDS patient, where there was very little immune function to prevent its growth.

Such situations allow viruses to grow far better than when they are confronted by a functional immune system. Suppression of the immune system is increasing. Immunosuppressive drugs are used in transplantation. Infection with HIV produces a long-lasting and major immunosuppression, and there are over 30 million cases worldwide. Some drugs of abuse such as anabolic steroids suppress the immune system.

There is convincing evidence that exposure to many of the chemicals used in modern life can induce immunosuppression. High levels of pesticides can enter rivers in runoff from agricultural land, along with other chemicals. They flow down into the sea, where they enter the marine food chain. As always, predators at the top of the chain accumulate high levels of such chemicals, and these have been linked to many outbreaks of disease in such animals, notably the European "seal plague" of 1988. This killed many thousands of seals and was identified as being caused by a novel virus related to both human measles and, more closely, to distemper virus of dogs. Although a novel virus was involved, the link to pesticides has been made many times. Seals are a predator, eating a mixed diet of other animals and accumulating any poisons the animals they eat are carrying. So are humans.

Until quite recently, even if a virus established itself within the human population and caused disease, it could remain restricted to a few hosts or one area. However, it is very unlikely that there are any truly unexplored areas left on this planet. Amplification of a virus by population movements has happened many times. In the case of HIV, the opening up of central Africa to trade and travel by the construction of the continent-spanning road known as the Kinshasa Highway has been blamed for bringing the virus out of central Africa. It is thought that HIV may have been present in rural areas there for some time before transmission to urban areas and into "amplifier" populations. The movement of people along the highway was the key.

To paraphrase the 19th century writer Robert Ingersoll, in nature there is no right or wrong; there are only consequences. It is always difficult to talk objectively about differing sexual morality, but it is a fact that prostitution in Africa and elsewhere is responsible for much of the heterosexual spread of HIV in those locations. However, prostitution can be necessary to survival when all other routes to get money are closed off. The problem of heterosexual AIDS in these countries is enormous, with such activity as a major route of transmission. The lack of resources for health care, particularly the reuse of hypodermic needles, gives the virus another amplification.

AIDS first came to global attention with the outbreak in the gay community in the United States. Amplified by practices that were common at that time, once it was established in this population, the virus exploded. High promiscuity was combined with "damaging" practices that allow direct contact of body fluids with blood.

Alongside this was a large group of intravenous drug abusers who were generally unwell, living in unsanitary conditions, injecting themselves with mixtures of drugs and unknown chemicals using needles contaminated with the blood of previous users. Another amplifier.

With these two groups to prey upon, HIV rates increased so rapidly that some groups, unaware of basic epidemiology, predicted that everyone on the planet would have the virus within a few years. This is obviously not the case. While the rate of increase has slowed, however, these amplifiers allowed it to establish a firm hold on the human race.

The biggest amplifier of infectious disease is, and will remain, poverty. Many viruses are transmitted by the fecal–oral route: contamination of food or drinking water with sewage. In developed countries, we take for granted our access to clean, safe drinking water. We are unusual, however, and in the crowded slums around the cities of the developing world, such viruses circulate and amplify to horrifying levels. In the most extreme cases, the sprawling refugee camps that rise up wherever there is conflict, even diseases we like to think of as only of historical interest will rise up and kill.

Such places, with crowded, unhygienic living conditions, poverty, and loss of the rules that govern established societies, are hothouses for disease. The new plagues of mankind may well come from the hidden places; the rainforest, the desert, the deep recesses of the world. However, it is in these hives of humanity that they will establish themselves most easily.

Sometimes efforts to help only make things worse. For example, the medical aid brought to the back country of Africa by missionary hospitals is vital. Working in horrifying conditions, the devoted individuals running these monuments to charity are saving lives every hour of every day, but sometimes things go wrong, like they did with Ebola.

Named for a river near the site of the original outbreak, Ebola is seen by many as the ultimate "killer virus." In some forms it kills up to 9 out of 10 people infected, almost liquefying the organs of the body in the most extreme form of the hemorrhagic fever. However, it is not a virus that is easily spread. In societies lacking even the most basic of medical care, victims would die but the virus would not spread far. However, if the victim is taken to a local hospital, one that has to reuse needles, that cannot afford to isolate patients or to sterilize equipment, the hospital itself acts as a focus for infection. As with the AIDS virus, attempts to help end up killing. Again, poverty is the killer.

OUT OF THE DARKNESS

While the deadly Ebola virus and its close relative, Marburg, attract a lot of attention and are assumed to come from an animal host deep in the African jungles, we do not actually know what their natural host is. They cause dramatic diseases, and so it would seem that they cannot circulate unseen in humans. As always, however, there must be a note of caution in saying something cannot happen. About 1 in 20 people in Zaire show the antibodies that mark previous infection, many times more than those who develop the disease. Does this mean that many get the virus but not the disease? If so, it could circulate in humans very well indeed. Or does it mean that there are also viruses circulating, like the Ebola Reston strain, that kill monkeys but are harmless in humans? We do not know the answer to this question either.

These lethal viruses appear from their unknown source, slay, and are gone. For a long time, bats have been suspected as the source, but this has never been proved, despite very intensive searches by many different agencies. So even the most dangerous viruses can remain mysterious.

VIRUS HUNTERS

It is becoming increasingly clear to governments and to the public that monitoring the appearance and frequency of infectious diseases is an essential part of disease control and that surveillance in developing countries is an essential part of any such program. The U.S. Senate Foreign Operations Subcommittee noted that "There is an urgent need . . . to significantly augment international surveillance and control mechanisms, and to strengthen the ability of developing countries, where deadly viruses often first gain a foothold, to protect and care for their people."

The process of identifying new or emerging diseases involves work at all levels, from the "disease cowboy" trying to find an outbreak, whose biggest problem may be where to find spare parts for his Jeep, to the molecular biologist compiling genetic information who may know almost nothing about the source of the disease or the people it kills. With the new molecular techniques now available, we have a far greater ability to identify new viruses, but knowing which will be the killers is still beyond us.

While we now know of many hundreds of viruses infecting humans, it is clear that many more remain to be discovered. Many of these will cause only mild disease, since those that cause obvious symptoms tend to be the first to be noticed. However, there are also a range of "orphan" diseases for which a cause has not yet been found. Until 1976, no cause had been identified for hemorrhagic fever with renal syndrome in Asia, a disease that had been known for over a thousand years. Now, we know it as the first of the hantaviruses. It would not be the last.

12

COUSINS
· · · · · · · · · · · · · · · ·

How can the skin of rat or mouse hold
Anything more than a harmless flea?
> RUDYARD KIPLING, *Natural Theology*
· ·

A horizon is nothing save the limit of our sight.
> ROSSITER WORTHINGTON RAYMOND
· ·

Sin Nombre virus was a big surprise. It was a new virus and a unique disease, but not for long.

OUTSIDE THE FOUR CORNERS

In June 1993, a 58-year-old Texas woman was the first victim to be identified outside of the Four Corners states. She developed the symptoms of the new disease, dying soon afterward. Testing at the CDC confirmed hantavirus infection, but she had not traveled outside eastern Texas for 3 months. It appeared that the disease was not confined to the Four Corners.

Then it showed up in Nevada. On June 7, a 24-year-old developed the disease. The next month, a 51-year-old woman contracted it. Both survived. California had a case in July in the Sierra Nevadas, a 27-year-old biologist living in a cabin with heavy rodent infestation. Another occurred in September, a 29-year-old ranch hand on the coast. Both cases were fatal. Then Oregon. Then North Dakota.

Suspicious cases from previous years were investigated using stored samples. Hantavirus infections were confirmed by the new tests all the way back to 1990. Most of those were outside the Four Corners: South Dakota, Kansas, Idaho, and Wisconsin.

During 1993, the Four Corners states accounted for three-quarters of the cases. The Four Corners was the center, but it was very clear that the "new" disease was neither new nor limited to the Four Corners.

Then the picture grew more complicated: American hantaviruses, causing pulmonary disease, that were not Sin Nombre.

BAYOU

The first sign came just over a month after the first cases in the Four Corners, in June 1993, with the death of a Louisiana bridge inspector from hantavirus pulmonary syndrome. When the genes of the virus were tested, they were something new: another hantavirus.

There were big differences to Sin Nombre in the genes and also in the disease. It was HPS, but it damaged the kidneys and caused hemorrhages. Sin Nombre didn't, but the Asian hantaviruses did. The new virus was named Bayou virus, and it seemed to have features from the Old World as well as the New World.

The next thing to be proved was that deer mice were not the only American rodent with a killer hantavirus. The natural range of the deer mouse is a huge region of North America, but it does not extend into the deep South. The host of Bayou virus was identified as the rice rat, *Oryzomys palustris*. Rice rats live clear across the South.

In 1995 and 1996, two more cases of Bayou HPS were seen. Both were in Texas, although one man seemed to have brought his virus from Louisiana. The other seemed to be a real Texas native.

All of the Bayou HPS cases had kidney damage. Sometimes Old World hantaviruses target the lung. Now a New World hantavirus was targeting the kidney. They seemed not to be that different after all, at least some of the time.

BLACK CREEK CANAL

Bayou was not the only cousin. On October 22, 1993, a 33-year-old Florida man was admitted to hospital with HPS, with the unusual addition of kidney problems. Bayou again? No. It was another new hantavirus. It was named Black Creek Canal hantavirus and is a relative of Bayou and Sin Nombre, but a new virus.

The cotton rat, *Sigmodon hispidus,* lives across a huge range from the southeastern United States down to South America. Of 90 cotton rats trapped in the area, 12 had antibody to the new virus. Another rodent, another hantavirus. Black Creek Canal virus has now been found in rats in four states, and rodent exterminators say the species is moving north. There has been only one case to date, and no deaths, but it is out there.

NEW YORK 1

Hantavirus disease seemed to cover almost all of the United States, with Bayou and Black Creek Canal filling in the largest gap, the deep South. The northeastern seaboard seemed to be a safe haven, until January 18, 1994.

On that day a 22-year-old man arrived at a Rhode Island emergency room with fever and muscle aches. He was discharged. Two days later he was back and this time, he was admitted. He died within 5 hours.

His blood had antibodies that reacted with Sin Nombre hantavirus, but he had not been out of the Northeast for 2 months. He had caught it locally.

Genetic testing showed a virus very much like Sin Nombre, but just different enough to be a new hantavirus. After a lot of searching, the investigators finally found infected mice living around the family holiday home on a rural vacation island at the eastern end of Long Island. They were not deer mice: they were *Peromyscus leucopus,* the white-footed mouse. It is a close relative of the deer mouse, so close that it is known to be able to carry Sin Nombre virus. It doesn't have as wide a range as the deer mouse, but it does live all across the northeast, and it seemed to have its very own hantavirus.

The new virus is related more closely to Sin Nombre than are the rat viruses that cause HPS, but is different enough to have its own name. Yet again the naming of this virus was to prove more difficult than it might have been. Trying to name it after the vacation island where the first case was infected was as unpopular as early attempts to give Sin Nombre a geographically exact name. Eventually a name was agreed upon. Even though it was found 80 miles from New York City, the new virus was named New York 1.

The idea that New York 1 was Sin Nombre that had switched to another mouse in "historically recent" times was raised. It was backed up when New York 1 was found to cause damage to the lungs of white-footed mice. Although this finding has been challenged, it may be evidence that this virus is still settling into its new host.

The new virus killed again in April 1995. Again, the infection happened in rural Long Island, at the victim's home.

MONONGAHELA

More support for New York 1 being new to its host came when a "missing link" virus showed up in deer mouse samples from a subspecies native to West Virginia. It was named Monongahela virus, and its genes look like it might be the halfway stage from Sin Nombre to New York 1.

Now it was clear that deer mice, already responsible for almost all of the HPS seen in the United States, carry at least two hantaviruses. Monongahela is not known to cause human disease. Yet. However, a case of HPS contracted in West Virginia showed more kidney damage than is usual for Sin Nombre. Added to that, Monongahela may just be the first sign of a hantavirus moving host. If they can do it once, they can do it again.

AND THE REST

As well as the killers, there are the "harmless" hantaviruses, and more are identified with each passing year. When an expert is asked about the potential of these viruses to kill, the answer is that human disease is "not documented," not "does not happen," just "not documented."

There are quite a few of these hantaviruses: for example, Isla Vista virus hantavirus, carried by the California vole, *Microtus californicus,* and Bloodland Lake hantavirus, carried by the prairie vole, *Microtus ochrogaster.* Both are related to the apparently harmless Prospect Hill hantavirus. Hantaviruses carried by voles seem to be the least harmful kind. So are they worrying? Maybe not. Maybe.

However, there are others about which it is less easy to relax: El Moro Canyon hantavirus, carried by the western harvest mouse, *Reithrodontomys megalotis;* and Muleshoe hantavirus, another doubling up, carried by the cotton rat, *Sigmodon hispidus,* that already provides a home to Black Creek Canal hantavirus.

Are these harmless? Don't bet on it.

El Moro Canyon hantavirus is a relative of Sin Nombre. It just happens to infect a different mouse, most of the time—a mouse that does not seek out human-built structures the way the deer mouse does, but all it takes is one mouse.

Muleshoe is a relative of Bayou. Sin Nombre and Bayou are both killers. Hantaviruses living in this type of rodent have a dark history.

SIN NOMBRE

The tests used in some cases would not have identified any of the "other" HPS hantaviruses as different. As far as we know, of the 196 cases of HPS reported to October 1998, Sin Nombre accounted for all but six.

The original is still out there and is still the worst, or at least the worst in North America.

SOUTH AMERICA

The isthmus of Panama looks narrow on a map of the world, but it is plenty wide enough for a mouse, or even a lot of mice, and it has been linking the continents for 6 million years.

BRAZIL

In 1994 the first cases of HPS were recognized in South America. In that year, three brothers living in the Juquitiba region of Sao Paulo State developed HPS, and two died. Their home was heavily infested with rodents.

Surveys in the area showed that up to 8% of people in the area had antibodies to hantavirus, which is high compared to the 2% seen across Europe or the less than 1% in the United States. Clearly there is a high level of the virus in the rodent host in the area. However, no infected rodents have yet been found, and the identity of the host is unknown.

There have been at least 11 cases of HPS in Brazil, and the death rate is very high, with over 80% of reported cases dying. This probably reflects the level of medical care combined with late identification of the disease, but may also mean that the Brazilian hantaviruses are unusually lethal. At least one case has shown the kidney problems that are unusual in most HPS.

The virus has been named Juquitiba, but it is not even known whether all of these cases are caused by the same virus.

Brazil is a huge country, accounting for almost half of South America. The back-country areas are remote and likely to contain many rodents, as yet unidentified, which could act as hosts for hantaviruses. It is also likely that many cases of HPS go unidentified. Compared to the situation in the United States or even in other South American countries, Brazil remains shrouded in uncertainty.

ARGENTINA

The picture in Argentina is very different. Argentina has a big problem with hantavirus, and they know it.

Six different hantaviruses have been named, four of which are known to cause human disease. Whether these really are different is still uncertain. There have been at least 115 cases since 1987, with a death rate of over 50%. Antibodies to hantaviruses are seen in between 1.5 and 15% of the population.

There seem to be three distinct areas of the country where HPS is seen. In the far northwest, in the sugar cane growing area of Orán, more than 30 cases have been identified. The hantavirus responsible seems to live in the long-tailed pygmy rice rat, *Oligoryzomys longicaudatus,* locally known as the *colilargo* (long-tailed) mouse. It has been named Oran virus.

In the center of the country, close to the capital, Buenos Aires, four different hantaviruses have been identified, carried by a variety of mice and rats: Lechigunas, Hu39694, Maciel, and Pergamino. Just to add to the brew, a kidney disease associated with hantavirus infection has been reported in the area, raising the possibility of Seoul virus infection carried by brown (or black) rats.

The first Argentinian hantavirus to be identified was in the southeast of the country. Samples from a fatal HPS case showed differences in its genes to those from known hantaviruses. Although the virus was related to North American hantaviruses, particularly Bayou and Black Creek Canal, it was new. Like Oran, it was carried by the long-tailed pygmy rice rat. It was named for the mountain range that runs through western Argentina: Andes virus.

It was with Andes virus that a nightmare became reality.

EL BOLSON

El Bolson is a small town of 15,000 inhabitants, lying in a wooded valley among the foothills of the Andes Mountains in southwest Argentina. The resort country around the town is a long way from the common image of rural South America. It is a popular vacation destination for the wealthy of Buenos Aires, a prosperous area dotted with cabins and holiday homes, with the local economy heavily dependent on tourism.

In 1996, there seemed to be no increase in the numbers of rodents in the area, but droughts and fires forced the local rodents to look for alternative food supplies, and they found them in the cabins. These rodents included *colilargo* mice.

The first to die was 41-year-old Rogelio Nassif, on September 26, 1996. On October 18, Esther Cortizo de Nassif, Rogelio Nassif's mother, died of the same infection. Clusters of the disease are often seen in families, living in the same conditions, but something new and terrifying was happening in El Bolson.

Rogelio Nassif's housekeeper, Flora Carriman, already showing the signs of the disease that was to kill her, attended the funeral of her employer's mother. Between 11 and 29 days later, all three people who traveled with her in the funeral car developed HPS.

It was known from cases in the United States that rodent nests in cars can be sources of infection. The Argentine health authorities tore the car to pieces looking for nests, but there were none. The only source of hantavirus in that car was Flora Carriman. The Andes virus was spreading between humans.

On October 21, Mother's Day, Dr. Roberto Martín, the physician who had attended Rogelio Nassif, died of HPS. Dr. Sergio Whisky, the principal of El Bolson hospital, had also attended the Nassif family. Fourteen days after his last visit to the Nassif home, he developed a fever. Three days later, hantavirus infection was confirmed. Dr. Whisky survived his fight with the Andes virus.

However, the spread of the virus was not over. Dr. Martin's wife, also a doctor, developed HPS. She survived, but two doctors who attended her, one in El Bolson and one in Buenos Aires, also developed the disease. Dr. Adriana Moreno de González died on December 2, 1996.

In the El Bolson outbreak, of 18 cases, 9 were to die. Five of the victims were doctors.

In the words of a Susana Cornaglia, a local fruit grower, "We thought it was an illness of poor people, an illness of dirt. This gave us a tremendous clap in our faces .... There was panic."

That panic was spread to the whole country by the press reaction. The nightmare that had been lurking since the Four Corners outbreak in 1993 was happening, over 5000 miles away from the Four Corners. A hantavirus could be passed on by infected humans and kill.

The nightmare, however, would come to an end. Dr. Paula Padula, chief of the Virology Department of the Carlos Malbran Institute in Buenos Aires, summed it up: "It is still not known whether the contagion was airborne or through body fluids.

Evidently the primary reservoir of the disease is the rodent, and the human chain of infection dies out." Sometimes luck is on our side, or at least it has been so far.

History repeats itself, and diseases are bad for local residents in more ways than one. In 1996, after the publicity surrounding the hantavirus outbreak, 90% of the tourists booked to travel to El Bolson canceled. The economy was hard hit, and the reaction of local people to the press coverage was like that in the Four Corners, 3 years before. They were angered over the panic about El Bolson, while there was almost no comment on cases in the north of the country, and repeated claims that the media had invented horror stories of chaos in El Bolson.

At the end of 1996, the president of Argentina and his entire cabinet traveled to El Bolson to reassure visitors. President Menem commented "I didn't see any mice during my stay." It still took a full year for the local economy to recover.

MORE BAD NEWS

Argentina had another problem not seen in the United States: HPS in Argentina is not as selective about causing disease.

HPS has been described as "another cause of adult respiratory distress syndrome." There are differences, but Sin Nombre HPS shares one feature of ARDS: it strikes adults. The youngest recorded case of Sin Nombre HPS was 11 years old. Cases below 16 years of age are rare. This is common with hantavirus disease, including the Eurasian versions. They seem to affect adults, with disease in children being rare and usually mild, but there are exceptions. Argentina is one.

Of five cases in children under the age of 12, three died. The youngest were only 5 years old. Obviously, South American hantaviruses are different.

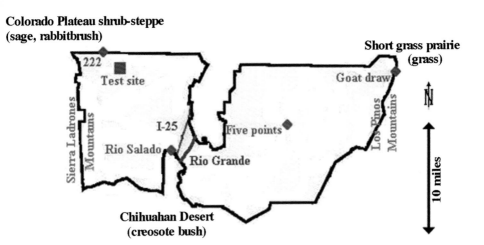

The Sevilleta National Wildlife Refuge spreads out around the valley of the Rio Grande like a butterfly, with wing tips resting on the flanking mountain ranges. Rodent numbers used in 1993 were assessed at several sites around the refuge covering a variety of terrain types. In the far northwest of the refuge is the remote site where new experimental enclosures are being constructed to study transmission and carriage of the virus among deer mice in near-natural conditions.

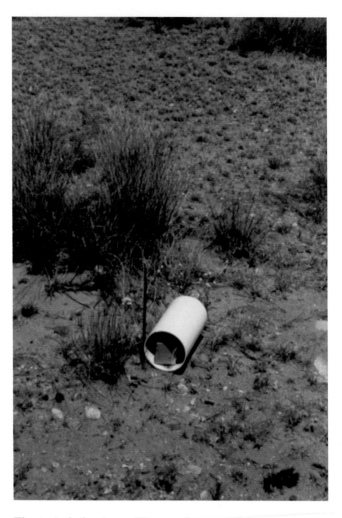

The typical aluminum "Sherman" trap used by investigators to collect rodents. The white plastic pipe acts as a sunshield. Traps are baited with rolled oats or other tempting rodent edibles, and a door snaps down behind the entering rodent, trapping it until a collector arrives. Sometimes a coyote gets there first, and the condition of some traps is a telling testament to the determination of a hungry coyote.

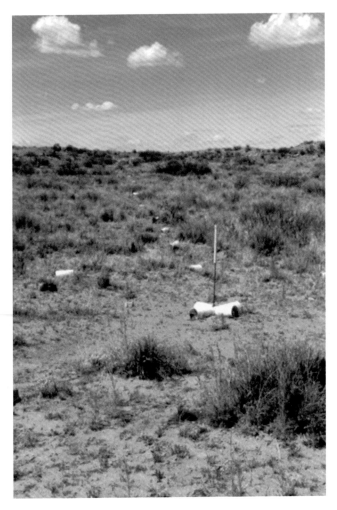

Traps are not used singly. Instead, a "trapping web" of 148 traps is used, with 12 lines of traps radiating out from a central point, covering a 200-meter-wide circle. Each web traps rodents from an area twice the size of the web. This allows the density of rodents to be determined more reliably than the use of isolated traps.

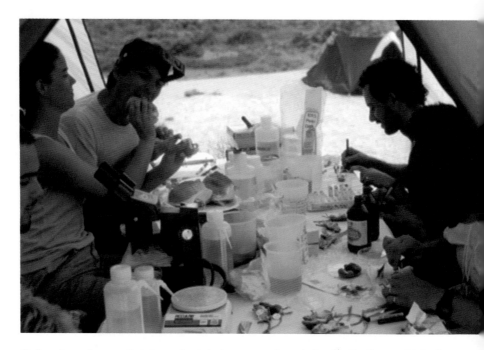

Before it was known that the rodents being trapped carried a deadly disease, biologists were quite happy to work with the rodents wearing no more than normal clothes. This "kitchen table" approach was to change dramatically after 1993. However, as Dr. Robert Parmenter observed, none of his 50 workers over a period of more than 10 years had contracted the new disease: "It was a hard disease to catch." In one survey, less than 1 in 100 people who worked closely with rodents had signs of exposure to the virus.

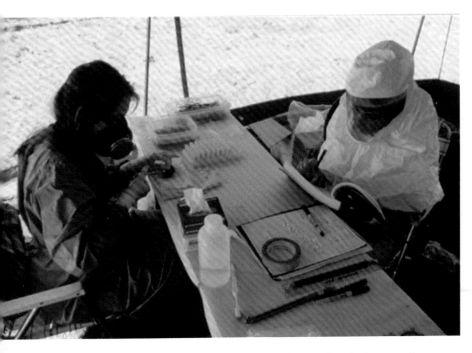

Since the identification of rodents as carriers for hantaviruses, the clothing used to carry out rodent surveys looks more like a space suit than ordinary clothes. The helmet or respirator protects the worker from breathing any dust or droplets, whereas the suit and gloves protect against splashes and allow the clothes underneath to remain free of potentially contaminated dust.

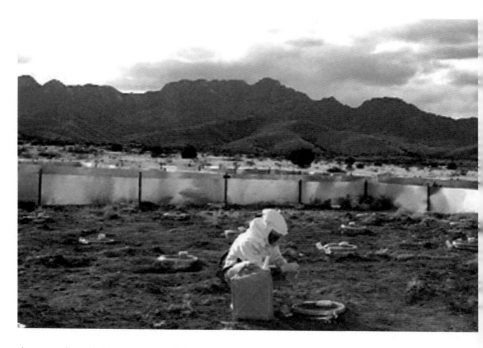

A protective suit in use at one of the quarantine enclosures on the Sevilleta National Wildlife Refuge south of Albuquerque. The round disks are wire mesh across the tops of "mouse nests." Each is made of two nested 5-gallon buckets inside a steel trashcan. The space between the buckets is filled with cotton wadding, forming the nest, with a 1-inch pipe leading down into it to allow mice to enter. The upper bucket is filled with dirt, insulating the next from extreme temperatures. The outer fence is 3 feet high and is made of steel plates that extend 2 feet below ground level. All of this is necessary to allow work with mice infected with lethal hantaviruses to be carried out in safety.

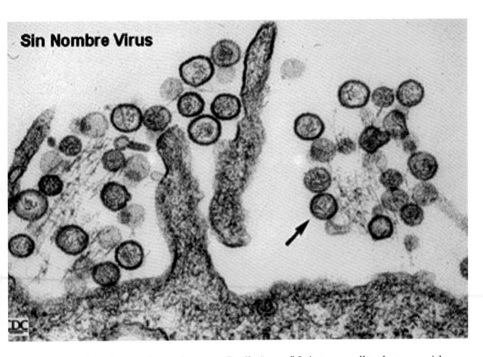

Sin Nombre Virus

In the fall of 1993, the new hantavirus was finally "seen." It is too small to be seen with any microscope using visible light. Instead an electron beam is used to look at an ultrathin section of an infected cell stained with electron-blocking heavy metals. The image is magnified over 100,000 times by the electron microscope. The new hantavirus is seen as dark-outlined circles (arrow).

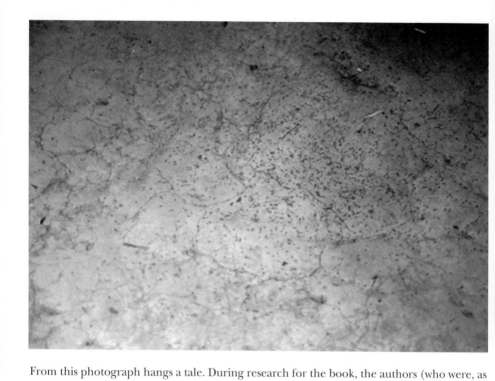

From this photograph hangs a tale. During research for the book, the authors (who were, as you might expect, well aware of the causes of hantavirus disease) were visiting a site where rodent surveys were carried out during the 1993 outbreak. The deer mouse (*Peromyscus maniculatus*) is found frequently at the site, which is at the altitude level where the Sin Nombre virus seems to be most common. At the time that this photograph was taken in April 1998, the site had only just opened to the public. The grass was still flattened by the recently melted snow, and the abandoned buildings there had been closed over the winter. The danger in "entering or cleaning rarely used, rodent-infested structures" was well known to us, but we still entered several buildings and structures at the site. Then, we entered this structure. Apparently no different to others on the site, there was no sign that it had been used to store anything of interest to rodents. As our eyes adjusted to the dim light, we realized that the scatter of small black dots on the floor was a liberal sprinkling of mouse droppings. Despite knowing the danger, our curiosity was enough that we remained to take this salutary photograph. This episode provides a graphic demonstration of the risks that even an informed individual can face. The first encounter with the potentially lethal environment was unexpected, as it is always likely to be. While few such encounters lead to disease, the potential for exposure to a lethal virus was all too real.

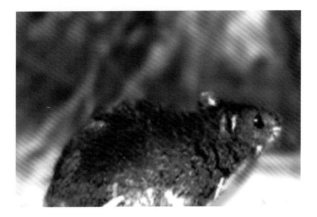

The rice rat (*Oryzomys palustris*) has soft gray-brown fur on its upper side and is paler underneath with very pale feet. Its body and head are about 5–6 inches long and has up to 7 inches of tail. They live in marshy areas and are often found in the water. They can breed for up to 10 months of the year, producing an average of four pups a month. The rice rat carries Bayou hantavirus.

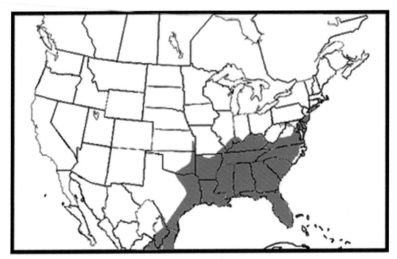

Range of the rice rat *(Oryzomys palustris)*

The range of the rice rat is more restricted than that of the cotton rat, but it still covers most of the southern states where deer mice are not found.

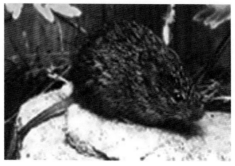

The cotton rat (*Sigmodon hispidus*) is definitely not cute. The fur is long and coarse and is buff gray and black on top with paler fur underneath. With a body and head 5–8 inches long and a tail 3–6 inches long, there can be over a foot of rat. There can also be many rats. Every year the cotton rat can have nine litters, usually of 5–6 pups, although up to 12 is known. Pregnancy lasts 4 weeks, and young rats can breed when they are 6 weeks old. In the wild, the cotton rat lives about a year, in burrows or nests in overgrown areas of grass and shrubs. The cotton rat carries Black Creek Canal hantavirus in Florida and Muleshoe hantavirus in west Texas. It has been suggested that cotton rats in the southern states and those from Texas southward all the way to Venezuela are actually different species, which would fit with the carriage of the two viruses.

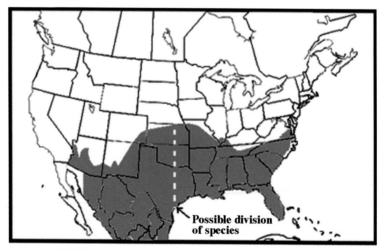

Possible division of species

Range of the cotton rat *(Sigmodon hispidus)*

The cotton rat very neatly covers most of that part of the United States where deer mice are not found. Only one case disease caused by Black Creek Canal hantavirus has been identified, and there is little information on the distribution of the virus outside Florida, but it does seem to be concentrated in small areas within the range of the cotton rat. West of the line, cotton rats may belong to a different species and have been identified as carrying Muleshoe hantavirus, which has not yet been associated with human disease.

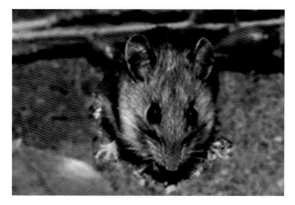

The white-footed mouse (*Peromyscus leucopus*) is a close relative of the deer mouse. It is slightly larger, with a body and head 3–4 inches long and a tail, (bicolored like that of the deer mouse) that is usually shorter than the rest of the mouse at 2–4 inches long. Its upper fur is brown and is generally paler than that of the deer mouse. Its underside and feet are white. It generally lives in wooded and brushy areas, although sometimes it will live in more open ground. It breeds less rapidly than the deer mouse and the young take longer to mature. The virus that it carries, New York 1 hantavirus, seems to be closely related to the Sin Nombre virus carried by the deer mouse.

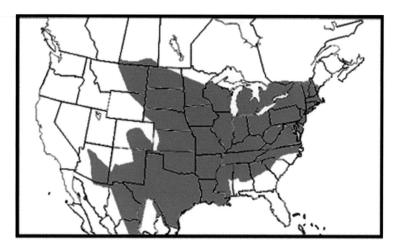

Range of the white-footed mouse (*Peromyscus leucopus*)

The range of the white-footed mouse, while not as large as that of the deer mouse, covers the northeastern seaboard where deer mice, cotton rats, and rice rats are not found.

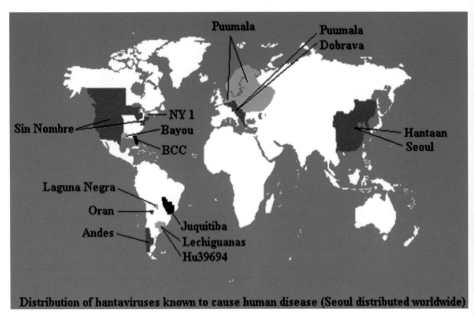

Distribution of hantaviruses known to cause human disease (Seoul distributed worldwide)

Hantaviruses are found on every continent except Antarctica, due to the worldwide presence of rats carrying the Seoul virus. Areas where hantaviruses are established and present at high levels (endemic) are shown on the map. Some sources suggest that hantaviruses extend across Europe and Asia, joining the Asian and European areas shown, but hard data on this are lacking. In some areas, multiple hantaviruses circulate. In the Americas, while relatively small areas are shown for the South American hantaviruses, these areas are likely to expand as further studies are carried out. No endemic hantaviruses have been identified yet in Australia or Africa, although hantavirus was suggested as one possible (if unlikely) cause for a recent outbreak of lethal pneumonia in southern Sudan.

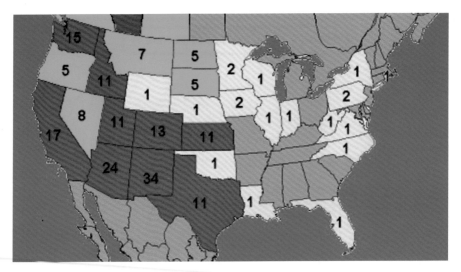

A map showing the state of origin of all cases of hantavirus pulmonary syndrome identified up to mid-October 1998 within the United States (colors indicated for Canada are accurate until the start of 1998). It is likely that areas outside of the Four Corners, where there is a high level of awareness, that some cases are being missed. All of the 48 contiguous states lie within the range of a rodent known to carry a hantavirus causing human disease. Cases have been seen in 29 of the 48 states. Even those states not reporting any cases to date are unlikely to be free of the viruses. Hantavirus disease is a national concern, not one restricted to the Four Corners.

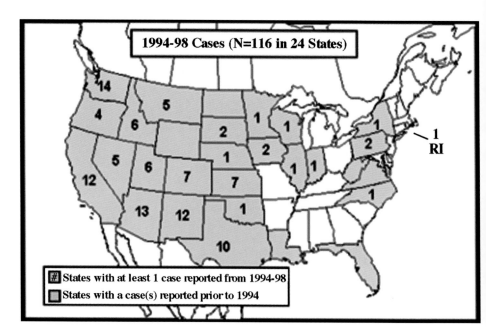

1994-98 Cases (N=116 in 24 States)

States with at least 1 case reported from 1994-98

States with a case(s) reported prior to 1994

Since the 1993 outbreak (which ran on for several months into 1994) until the possible outbreak in 1998, the Four Corners area ceased to be the main focus of hantavirus pulmonary syndrome within the United States. The highest number of cases since the start of 1994 has actually been in Washington state in the Pacific Northwest, possibly reflecting different weather patterns in years not affected by the El Niño phenomenon. While hantavirus disease is still predominantly a disease of the western half of the country, cases are seen in all regions.

IMMUNOPATHOLOGY

HPS kills because of the immune response to the virus. It is an immunopathological disease, where the workings of the immune system itself produce the disease.

Why this virus produces such a massive immune response is unknown. There are some proteins, superantigens, that act directly on the immune system. Both bacteria and viruses can make such proteins, which can produce massive immune activation. It seems that in Sin Nombre there might be something like this. Whatever it is, it pushes the immune system into killing the body that gave it birth.

A specialized form of immunopathology also exists where the immune system attacks the body directly, known as autoimmune disease. One part of the immune system known to be involved with an autoimmune disease: the HLA molecules.

Whether the same mechanisms are involved in producing the severe form of HPS seen with HLA-B*35 is unknown. However, a mechanism may be waiting to be found, and maybe, just maybe, there will then be some way to stop it.

There is another effect resulting from the role of the body's own immune system in HPS. At best, antiviral drugs can stop a virus in its tracks, blocking it completely. However, by the time the symptoms of HPS are seen, the virus is blocked, with the whole disease caused by the immune system's reaction to the infection. As a result, no antiviral drug is going to control the disease once it has reached this stage. Controlling the mind-numbing complexities of the immune system is still at the same level as kicking a television set to see if that makes it work any better.

What can be done?

14

HOW TO STOP
A VIRUS
· · · · · · · · · · · · · ·

There is no miracle drug to cure HPS
· ·

An ounce of prevention is worth a pound of cure
BENJAMIN FRANKLIN
· ·

There were 196 identified cases of hantavirus pulmonary syndrome up to October 1998. Throughout the New World—North and South America—at least 200 more cases have been seen up to that date.

Many articles have been written praising the speed of the work that identified Sin Nombre in 1993 and just how important modern techniques were. As Dr. C. J. Peters said in his book, "Virus Hunter," "It was the shortest amount of time ever needed to identify a virus during an outbreak."

There is no denying the speed of the identification.

Why, however, are American hantaviruses still killing people? Science has brought paeans to the investigators, but what has it brought to the potential victims?

HOW TO STOP A VIRUS

There are four basic ways to stop a virus from killing people:

- Prevention: Stop it from infecting in the first place.
- Vaccination: Help the body to fight it off.
- Antiviral drugs: Stop the virus from growing.
- Medical care: Support the victims until they recover from the infection.

With Sin Nombre and other hantaviruses, only two out of four apply, even now.

HOLLYWOOD

The public perception of what happens once a disease is identified differs widely from reality. Accustomed to movies and television where all the loose ends are neatly tied up within the span of 2 hours, minus commercials, the public expects immediate results. It is easy to see why.

In the movie "Outbreak," a whole town is dying of a deadly new hemorrhagic fever. A brave military scientist (played by Dustin Hoffman, with definite elements of C. J. Peters) finds a monkey that has survived the new virus. Within a very short time (it has to be short, there is a plane on the way to bomb the whole town) all of the victims are saved, and the scientist's wife, who was near death from the disease, has her lip gloss back. Roll credits.

It doesn't happen that way.

Back in 1993, residents in the Four Corners believed that the CDC would soon announce a definitive diagnosis, followed shortly thereafter by a cure, and then everyone could go back to life as usual. In 1999, we have no vaccine, no antiviral drug. Why not?

THE SURVIVING MONKEY

This is a common element in movies. Once a survivor is found, monkey or human, everyone can relax. A cure is found.

This idea seems to have originated in "passive immunization," where antibodies extracted from the blood of an immune individual are given to potential disease victims to boost the immune response against that disease.

This method is widely used, for example, for chicken pox in the United Kingdom. However, it moderates disease rather than cures it. Even with the whole of the population to call upon, there is still a dire shortage of the antibody preparation. How one small monkey could provide enough antibody to protect an entire town was not specified.

Added to this, passive immunization has been used for Ebola hemorrhagic fever, the prototype for the movie, but the jury is still out whether it was of any use at all. Its use was more in desperation than for any real hope that it would protect.

In the case of hantaviruses, we know that they can persist in the rodent host for months, even for the life of the host. During this time the host is making antibodies, quite a lot of them. By the usual tests, they appear to be effective, but they are not. How the virus eludes them is unknown, but it does.

So a few antibodies are unlikely to turn the tide. Sadly, life is not like the movies.

What has been tried?

VACCINATION

A vaccine is first and foremost a way of preparing the immune system to fight off something it has never seen. Someone who has had an infection and recovered generates an immune response to the agent, whether it is a bacterium, a virus, or something else entirely. This immune response is often, but not always, protective. That is, if exposed to the same agent again, that individual will not usually develop as severe a disease. A vaccine looks like the agent, enough like it that the immune response to the vaccine is protective when the agent itself come along.

There are a number of ways to make a vaccine. (1) It can be a live version of the agent, weakened by adapting it to another host; the chicken pox vaccine is made this way. (2) It can be the agent, killed chemically, so that only the proteins are present to stimulate the immune response, like the rabies vaccine. (3) It can be some small part of the agent, most often one or more proteins. This only targets part of the agent, but if that part is selected carefully, it can be enough to protect.

If the vaccine is part of the agent, it can be purified from the agent itself, as with the influenza vaccine. Alternatively, the gene coding for it can be expressed, in bacteria or some other easily grown cell such as yeast, as is done to make the hepatitis B vaccine.

There are other methods, including putting the gene into a weakened form of another virus or even just into a replicating loop of deoxyribonucleic acid (DNA), but no vaccines made these ways are available yet.

HANTAVIRUS VACCINES

Several of these approaches have been tried for hantaviruses.

For the Asian Hantaan virus that causes the most severe form of Asian hantavirus disease, at least four vaccines have been developed. At the U.S. Army Medical Research Institute of Infectious Diseases in Maryland, a weakened form of the live virus smallpox vaccine was used, into which genes from Hantaan virus were inserted. The vaccine was tested in human trials in 1994 and 1995.

In China, different types of inactivated ("killed") Hantaan vaccines are being tested, along with vaccines that will also generate immunity against Seoul hantavirus. In Korea, "Hantavax" is a commercially available inactivated vaccine against Hantaan virus.

Some experimental vaccines exist against the European Puumala hantavirus, using Puumala virus protein joined to other proteins that simulate the immune system. A DNA-only vaccine is also being tested.

However, as yet there is no vaccine against any American hantavirus yet and there are major technical obstacles to any attempt to create one.

WHY NOT?

Some problems are purely technical, like the way the necessary gene of Sin Nombre virus contains codes that stop them from being easy to make in the normal types of cell. Others concern what kind of vaccine to make.

A vaccine can be designed to produce antibodies, to activate the killer cells of the immune system, or to do both. However, if the damage in HPS is caused by killer cells, then do you really want to activate those? Some vaccines only produce antibody and seem to be effective, but the virus can grow in mice with high levels of antibody present, so would antibody be enough? Nobody knows the answers.

Then there is the problem of how to test the vaccine. There is no animal system that develops anything like the human disease, so studies of protection against disease are not possible.

There is also the problem of assessing protection against HPS in humans. In China there are over 100,000 cases of hantavirus disease a year, but in the Americas 5 years of intensive study have identified only 400 cases. There is little doubt that many people would want the vaccine, but very few of those would actually develop HPS without it. So how can the protective effect of the vaccine be tested?

Some work is under way, including a DNA-only vaccine under development at the University of New Mexico, but the problems of testing any vaccine remain huge.

ANTIVIRAL DRUGS

Antiviral drugs have been slower and more difficult to develop than antibiotics for one major reason. Bacteria are living cells, unlike those in higher forms of life but still alive. They breathe, convert food to energy, assemble complex molecules from simple ones, and make more bacteria. Unlike bacteria, viruses cannot grow on their own. A virus is only a package of genetic information that reprograms a cell to make more viruses. As a result, most of the processes used by a virus are the same as those of the cell, and there are very few targets specific to the virus. Many candidate antiviral drugs fail in testing because they are harmful to the host cell, and even some of those in use have significant toxic effects.

RIBAVIRIN

As outlined in Chapter 4, ribavirin (Virazole) was made available for use during the 1993 outbreak in the Four Corners on the basis of its known effects against Hantaan virus in Chinese studies. Later work has shown that Sin Nombre is sensitive to ribavirin in isolated cells.

Although there was a decrease in deaths in patients treated with ribavirin, this was within the range of random chance. But ribavirin was used very late in the course of the disease. An international trial has been started at Albuquerque, New Mexico; Salt Lake City, Utah; Birmingham, Alabama, and Edmonton, Alberta, Canada, in which the drug is given as early as possible. The results are not yet available.

Ribavirin is not without its problems. First, it is only licensed in the United States to be given as an aerosol against a respiratory virus infection of children. Second, it is expensive and of very limited availability. Third, and most important, it has some very unpleasant side effects, including anemia, headache, respiratory depression, and even cardiac arrest. In the 1993 outbreak, 77% of those treated developed anemia, with 20% needing a blood transfusion. These are significant side effects.

Its use has been described as an "emotional gesture" rather than a medical treatment. When a trial was suggested in Argentina, home of the Andes virus, the most worrying of the American hantaviruses, it was reported that health-care professionals refused to use it.

Despite all that, at the University of New Mexico, ribavirin is kept for use in case a laboratory worker becomes infected with Sin Nombre virus. It is still in the CDC treatment protocol, and many physicians say they would use it if they or a family member contracted HPS. That doesn't mean it has been shown to work; it simply means ribavirin is still all there is to try. Sometimes any hope is better than none at all.

NEW DRUGS

There are no antiviral drugs under development against hantaviruses that are anywhere close to becoming available. Some work is under way on European and Asian viruses using components of the immune system, but early results have not been promising. For the American hantaviruses, the same problems for vaccines hold true: there is no animal system to allow testing and very few human cases, which progress very rapidly. Of course there is another problem: an antiviral drug has very little effect when the killer is the body's own immune system.

Rapid developments are unlikely, which leaves the other two elements: medical care of HPS cases and preventing infection in the first place.

PREVENTION

The single most important discovery in the history of Sin Nombre was that it is a hantavirus. Based on what was known about how hantaviruses infect humans in Asia and Europe, advice to avoid rodents was given. Studying rodents around where infection had happened identified the specific host, the deer mouse, which did not really change the advice to the public all that much. Telling people to creep up on suspicious rodents and check if they have the "terete, sharply bicolored tail" listed as characteristic of the deer mouse is not very practical.

On this subject, the Navajo have it right. *Na'atoosi* translates as "mouse." Not "deer mouse," "member of the genus *Peromyscus,*" or "member of the *Sigmodontinae.*" In the same way the long-tailed pygmy rice rat is commonly known in South America as the *colilargo* (long-tailed) mouse. Avoiding rodents is about as far as it goes.

In criticizing media coverage of the 1993 hantavirus outbreak in the Southwest, tourism professionals scoffed, "The only thing we have to fear is fear itself." In fact, the exact opposite may be true. Fear, or at least healthy caution, may be all we have to save us.

RISKS

When the cause of the new disease in the Four Corners was identified in 1993, there was a lot of worry about possible high numbers of cases that fall. This was because of the behavior of hantaviruses elsewhere. Hantaan in Asia and Puumala in Europe both show peaks of disease in the fall as rodents move into buildings in search of food and warmth, but the fall peak did not happen for Sin Nombre. In fact, the highest number of cases of Sin Nombre HPS seems to be in the late spring and early summer.

So Sin Nombre was following different rules. Studies were carried out to identify what those rules were. The most important thing to identify was precisely what activities increased the risk of Sin Nombre disease. It was no surprise when many of the risks were similar to those for Hantaan, but there were differences.

When looking at 17 of the first 21 cases, scientists from the CDC showed links to the number of rodents in or around a house. Where the disease occurred there tended to be more rodents. There was also a link with specific activities: cleaning food stores or agricultural outbuildings or tilling a garden. The final factor was a history of an illness with an immune system component, such as allergies or asthma. These are individuals whose immune systems are already quite active. No link to domestic animals was shown, although cats had been shown to increase risk in Asian hantaviruses.

A second study with a larger number of cases identified where 70 victims of the disease were likely to have become infected. Exposure to rodents in or around the house was by far the most common route, accounting for over two-thirds of cases (69%). Exposure only at work was much less likely to result in disease (4%). The rest of the cases had possible exposure in more than one situation, except for one group.

The letter reporting the study had the title "Hantavirus Pulmonary Syndrome Associated with Entering or Cleaning Rarely Used, Rodent Infested Structures." In 9% of cases this seemed to be the only risk, and details of six cases were given. Other similar cases came under the heading of domestic exposure, so this group is more significant than it would at first appear.

Since then there have been many cases where cleaning out buildings was the obvious risk. A pool pump house, a holiday cottage, a canning shed, and a stable were all sites of exposure.

Although more recent work has shown more occupational and recreational cases, this is why the CDC guidelines include so much advice on how to clean up any rodent debris, and it may also be why the number of cases of Sin Nombre HPS peaks in the late spring and early summer.

The time from exposure to virus to development of symptoms seems to be between 8 and 40 days. So if people are going to contract the disease spring cleaning outbuildings or closed up rooms or opening up summer residences, that would mean that most cases would occur just about when they do.

However, these are not the only risks.

Scientifically and anecdotally, there have been cases of HPS reported in which there were rodents living in a mattress, where rodents were nesting in a car ventilation system, where a mouse ran across the face of a camper, and where a single mouse nest was cleaned out of a window seat.

It is very difficult to be certain that any one event caused the infection because exposure to rodents or rodent-contaminated material is relatively common and often unnoticed. A mouse running over someone's face is a lot more memorable than sweeping up some sticks and straw. However, the single mouse on the face is most likely to be hantavirus free, even when an outbreak is under way, whereas a nest used by many mice is far more likely to contain the virus.

FINDING THE SOURCE

There are ways to track down the source of the infection. The same genetic methods that allowed the rapid identification of Sin Nombre can be used to look at the genes of a virus that has caused HPS. Rodents are trapped at possible sites where infection could have occurred and their genes are examined. Comparing the genetic code shows which are most like the virus from the human case. Even viruses that are of the same type will have some variation, usually well below that needed to call them a new virus. Viruses from different locations will have more variation.

The first time this method was used it allowed the site of infection to be identified in two-thirds of the cases studied. It is now used routinely to identify how and where an infection occurred. It is much more accurate, and sometimes more honest, than human recollection.

RECREATIONAL RISK

Many of the visitors to the deserts of the Southwest have been drawn there by the archaeological attractions, many of which are good habitat for small rodents. That sort of tourism involves poking one's nose into dark and dusty places. Archaeologists, logically, are at greater risk than tourists for several reasons. First and most importantly, they spend much more time in high-risk environments. They are more likely to enter sites that have not been disturbed recently and are more likely to engage in activities, such as excavation, that could stir up virus-laden rodent debris.

During the initial outbreak, archaeologists expressed concerns about the level of risk they might experience and guidelines were developed to protect them. To a mouse, after all, an ancestral Puebloan granary was no different than a 20th-century feed bin; both are dry places to store food. Experts debating the risk to archaeologists decided there was probably more risk from mice nesting on top of an excavation site than from anything dug out of the site.

As yet, there is almost no information on how stable the virus actually is outside its host rodent. Its genes are made of RNA, rather than the more stable DNA, and it is surrounded by a fragile fatty sheath, so it is relatively unstable compared to some other viruses, such as smallpox, for which there is real concern over disruption of centuries-old grave sites.

Pack rat middens have been found that are up to 40,000 years old, preserved by rat urine. After that amount of time, even that much urine is unlikely to have anything alive in it. There is likely to be an upper limit. However, there is almost no information on how long the virus remains able to infect when it is in a mouse nest. They need to be treated as dangerous at all times.

Although it's scientifically irresponsible to douse fragile relics with bleach, many other precautions may be taken, and thus far those safeguards have proven adequate. Neither professional nor amateur archaeologists have fallen victim to hantavirus, and the risk to other visitors seems slight as well—if only they exercise awareness and take sensible precautions. While the perception of risk is indeed a deterrent to tourism, there seems to be little evidence to suggest that hantavirus presents a substantial risk to visitors to the archaeological wonders of the Southwest.

EDUCATION

Public education is vital to prevention. Major education programs have been carried out in the United States, Chile, and other affected countries targeting likely areas for the disease. In the United States, a lot of effort has gone into educating the public in the Four Corners, including those on the Navajo reservation. Information has been prepared as leaflets, posters, and videos. However, one major problem is that people most likely to be exposed to rodents are those least likely to be reached by the information and are also those least likely to be able to act on the advice.

Isolated homes, language difficulties, or lack of access to health care can prevent information being received. For example, CDC educational material was initially not available in

Spanish. Once it was made apparent that Spanish speakers account for almost one-eighth of HPS cases, this was corrected. However, other factors still exist. Local education programs can be very effective at getting information across, but are far more difficult to organize than simply providing some leaflets or posters. They are also much more expensive.

A lack of resources or cultural attitudes can prevent information being acted upon even if people are informed. For example, Paraguayan Indians can be told time and again about risks, but if they cannot afford rodent-proof containers to store food in, they cannot act on well-intentioned advice to use such containers.

Education is working. Health-care workers have noted a huge shift in attitudes toward rodents in the American southwest. Among some groups, mice are regarded with far greater caution than they used to be. Dr. Brian Hjelle, who runs the hantavirus testing laboratory at the University of New Mexico, commented that calls to him during 1998 have shown this very clearly. He credits this with preventing an outbreak in the area in a year when all the conditions for an outbreak were in place.

A survey being run by Dr. Robert Parmenter of the Sevilleta research program is looking into the sales in selected towns in the Four Corners of bleach, gloves, and other materials that would be used if CDC guidelines were being followed. This of course, however, does not show whether they are being used just as precautions or whether they are going where they are really needed.

WARNINGS

How do people know when HPS is likely?

People on the ground can see the obvious increase in rodent numbers known as a "rodent bloom." They can also see when the land is greener than usual or when the piñon pines have more nuts than usual to provide winter food. If they are told that these are the signs warning of disease, they can take more care.

That is not enough for the organizations that need to have resources ready to deal with an outbreak before it happens. They need as much warning as they can get, and they will use any means they can to get it.

Orbiting the earth are thousands of artificial satellites, among them the Landsat survey satellites. First launched in 1972, the Landsats scan the Earth's surface in narrow color bands, some outside the range of the human eye. By combining images from different bands, images can be built up that show patterns relevant to geology or agriculture. In particular, the amount and growth of vegetation can be mapped. Because these satellites are permanently scanning the earth, automated monitoring for "dangerous" patterns can be set up.

One major study compared the sites of infection of 1993 HPS cases with Landsat images for the area. The conclusion was that vegetation was associated with disease risk, which was a fairly safe hypothesis from the very beginning.

So why are the satellite images needed? They may help catch new plant growth in sparsely settled areas and can be utilized by large organizations instead of a nationwide network of surveyors. The advantage came in showing patterns that might remain undetected on the ground, in being able to see the forest for the trees. Satellite information helps confirm the link between El Niño and Sin Nombre.

ELEMENTS OF PREVENTION

Prevention is avoiding rodents; keeping the home and out-buildings free of anything that might attract rodents; blocking any rodent entry points; using gloves and disinfectants when cleaning any area with rodent debris in it; avoiding dust; airing out newly opened buildings; and even encouraging outdoor predators such as owls, snakes, or coyotes. One coyote was discovered with 20 mice in its stomach. That can make a difference in a limited area.

These simple procedures are credited by at least one expert with having controlled an outbreak in the Four Corners during 1998. However, another expert noted that of the last six HPS patients he saw, all six claimed to have followed the guidelines. The risk may be just one deep breath of virus-laden air before the discovery of rodent detritus sends a cautious person running for a dust mask. It may be the failure to pinch the metal clip tightly against the nose. These are small details, not even errors in judgment, not mistakes, just a convergence of circumstances, but the result can be a disease that still kills a third of the people it infects.

However effective they are (or are not), these are the only currently available ways to control the disease. The full CDC guidelines are given in Appendix A.

MEDICAL CARE

Once HPS develops, there is no proven drug against the virus. All that is done is done to support the body and help it to survive while it fights off the infection. The initial signs of HPS are described in detail in Chapter 13, and individuals who experience these symptoms and who believe they might have been exposed to the virus are urged to contact their health-care provider immediately.

One reason for the improvement in the survival rate since 1993 is that patients are being identified more rapidly and as a result are reaching the hospital earlier. Once the patient reaches hospital, treatment may vary. The outline that follows is derived from guidelines on the CDC Hantavirus website. The original protocols were issued by the University of New Mexico Medical Center at Albuquerque, one of the most experienced at dealing with HPS, where Drs. Fred Koster, Howard Levy, and Mark Crowley are at the forefront of the battle against this killer.

This summary is given for general information only, and any interested clinicians should refer to the full guidelines, which are updated as new information becomes available.

All patients receive broad spectrum antibiotic coverage until HPS is proven (in case of bacterial infections such as pneumococcal pneumonia or pneumonic plague). Early intensive care management is important, with a prompt correction of electrolyte, pulmonary, and hemodynamic abnormalities.

Catheterization of the pulmonary artery is used for monitoring the heart. The UNM approach is to administer fluids and then to give inotropic drugs, which help the heart to contract more efficiently.

Cardiopulmonary support with extracorporeal membrane oxygenation (ECMO) has been evaluated. With ECMO, blood is removed from the body to be supplied with oxygen. ECMO used by doctors at UNM is credited by Dr. Koster with saving over half of the patients not otherwise expected to survive and is now used routinely at UNM in severe cases.

THE HEART

Dr. Koster has been involved with HPS since the earliest days; it was he and Dr. Levy who treated the first cases to reach Albuquerque in May 1993. Dr. Koster is currently campaigning to change the name of the disease from "hantavirus pulmonary syndrome" to "hantavirus cardiopulmonary syndrome," to recognize the key role of the heart. HPS floods the lungs, but the heart is damaged in multiple ways; strained by the failure of the lungs and poisoned by toxins. Shock and stress on the heart cause the rapid death that marks HPS. ECMO provides double support. It not only oxygenates the blood, but may also remove the toxins, protecting the heart and saving lives.

INTENSIVE CARE

As is obvious from a reading of the previous list, the patient stands a far better chance of survival in a hospital with good intensive care facilities, but there are other elements as well. Examination of the statistics for the Four Corners states shows a strong link with referral to a hospital with extensive experience in handling HPS. In the words of Dr. Koster, "This disease has a dramatic and precipitous course. You have to be at the bedside to appreciate that."

AFTERMATH

Following a bout with HPS, patients may recover fully, but some do not. One man whose exercise program used to consist of a 5-mile run every day and weight sessions three times a week could only walk 1 mile, three times a week, a year after HPS and after 6 months of intensive training. Other HPS patients report quicker recoveries, but the experience has a psychological aftermath as well.

WHERE HAS THE MONEY GONE?

In the wake of the events of early 1993, $6 million in additional federal funding was organized by the eight senators representing the Four Corners states. Since then, it has been hard to deny hantavirus research a hearty slice of the funding pie. When constituents are scared and noisy, politicians take notice.

So what has the money done? There is no vaccine, no drug, and no control for the host species, just gloves and bleach, as it was back in 1993.

Firstly, it should be noted that the actual amount spent on hantavirus research is still small compared to some other areas, such as AIDS research. And even there, we have drugs, but no vaccine. And prevention is still the best option.

Some money has gone overseas, particularly to South America to identify the problem there. This is not irrelevant. Could a stowaway group of *colilargo* mice establish a breeding colony north of the equator instead of south? It cannot be ruled out. Denver is the same distance from the equator as El Bolson and in the foothills of a mountain range with definite similarities to the Andes. It is very unlikely, but the Andes virus bears watching.

What about the money that has stayed in the United States?

There is no denying that some of the money has produced results. Money from the National Institutes of Health has supported valuable work, notably at UNM. Testing and identifying patients for early treatment have brought the death rate down. Public education is credited by at least one expert with having prevented a 1993-scale outbreak in 1998 and has undoubtedly saved lives. Outbreaks can be tracked, and the source of the virus identified. Hantaviruses are very difficult to work with, but despite that work at some centers has produced results.

But in the end, what people see is that a lot of apparently expensive scientific research has been done, but there is still no vaccine and no antiviral drug. Many scientists are employed. A lot of information has been gathered, and information is never worthless. It has been said that if the public does not understand science, then that is the fault of the scientist, not the public. For the taxpaying citizen, the question of exactly what the money has bought to make his or her life safer does seem to be going unanswered.

15

OUTBREAKS
· · · · · · · · · · · · · · · · · · · ·

It's not a big killer . . . More and more we will be seeing viruses that, even if they cause disease, infect only a few people in a few places . . . Sin Nombre is lethal, but it does not kill many people, and almost certainly never will

DR. BRIAN HJELLE,
in conversation with one of the authors
· ·

No man is an Island, entire of itself . . . any man's death diminishes me, because I am involved in Mankind. And therefore never send to know for whom the bell tolls; It tolls for thee.

JOHN DONNE, *Meditations XVII*
· ·

HANTAVIRUS NOW

The American hantavirus disease was first recognized in the spring of 1993. Up to the middle of October 1998, 196 cases of hantavirus pulmonary syndrome were recorded in the United States. Fifty-three of these were in 1993. Of all cases, most (61%) were male. This is common to hantaviruses, including those in Europe and at least some parts of Asia. Throughout the Americas, males also seem to be at greater risk of disease, accounting for 73% of cases in Chile, 60% in Argentina, and 67% in Canada.

Despite the early identification of HPS as a "Navajo disease," this is not how it has developed. By fall 1998, whites accounted for three-quarters of all cases (75%) and Native Americans for less than a quarter (22%). Even in 1993, Native Americans accounted for less than half of cases (49%).

NOT ALL PEOPLE ARE THE SAME

If the statistics for HPS are examined, there are some variations. As well as a lower frequency of disease in some populations who have been in an area for a long time, there are some differences common to hantaviruses generally.

One of the few good things about Sin Nombre HPS is that the disease does not seem to be seen in children. It also does not seem to affect the fetus in pregnant women except as a result of the illness it causes in the mother. In North America, HPS remains a disease of adults. The youngest case was 11 years old; the mean age to date is 37. Hantaan in Asia also shows this. The usual age for disease is 20 to 50 years, and when the disease is seen in children it is milder. Puumala in Europe is similar. With the single deadly exception of Andes, hantaviruses do not seem to cause severe disease in children.

Why?

The short answer is that we do not know. There are diseases seen only in adults. HPS itself was originally thought to be a form of an adult-specific condition; adult respiratory distress syndrome. Major changes take place in the body at puberty, not just on the outside. Some proteins on the surface of cells of the immune system are different after puberty. For a disease like HPS that involves the immune system as part of the disease itself, this could be key.

Work in Paraguay has produced some interesting clues. Up until puberty, children do not have antibody to the local hantavirus, Laguna Negra. In adults, 50% will have antibody by the age of 30, after which the figure rises no higher. Dr. Fred Koster of the University of New Mexico suggests that it could be that the 50% are all of the population that the virus is capable of infecting.

The recent discovery that some HPS viruses need a highly variable surface protein to be able to enter the cells of the body could provide a way for that to happen. It could be that the "uninfected" adults have been exposed to the virus, but do not have the particular protein it needs to even begin infection. Without that the virus cannot even grow enough to generate antibody against itself. If that protein was one that was only made at or after puberty, children would also not make antibody, no matter how many times they were exposed. It is an interesting idea, but unproven.

There is another difference in hantavirus infections. More men than women seem to get the disease in general. For HFRS in Korea, the ratio is two or three men to every woman. It is the same in Europe. It may be more even among some population groups, but the difference is real. Again, there are differences between the sexes at the biochemical level, but how this relates to the development of HPS, nobody knows.

IN THE FINAL ACCOUNTING

The death rate from HPS is still high. Overall, 44% of cases in the United States are fatal. Since 1993, improvements in care combined with the earlier identification of disease and recognition of milder cases have combined to reduce the death rate. In 1993, 60% died. Since January 1994, 34% have died. This is slightly higher than the death rate of 30% seen in Canada, but lower than Chile or Argentina, and far lower than Brazil.

Following 1993, there has been a movement away from the site of the initial outbreak. Overall, less than half (42%) of all cases have occurred in the Four Corners states (which do, of course, account for only 4 states out of 50, and pretty empty ones at that). However, with cases from 1994 to spring 1998, the percentage in the Four Corners States drops to 31%. In fact, the state with the highest number of cases since 1993 was Washington, with 14 cases.

Why?

EL NIÑO?

If the predicted effect of El Niño on different areas of the United States is examined, it is not uniform. The usual understanding of the effect of El Niño is of increased rainfall, but in fact the predicted rainfall is unchanged in many states, and the northwestern states are actually predicted to be drier.

One basic rule with hantaviruses seems to be that rain makes vegetation, vegetation makes mice, and mice make disease. This is a vast oversimplification, but it happened in the Four Corners in 1993 and in Paraguay in 1995. There were different causes in some outbreaks, but there is a definite link to rainfall.

So what happens when it is not an El Niño year?

The year 1993 was an El Niño year, and 64% of all cases were in the Four Corners states: 34 cases of 53. During 1993, the northwestern states of Washington, Oregon, Idaho, Montana, and Wyoming had just one case of HPS identified.

Then, from January 1994 to the spring of 1998, the Four Corners states had 30 cases and the northwestern states 29 cases. Better identification of the new disease undoubtedly accounts for some of that, but HPS was showing a very different pattern of infection.

During the spring and summer of 1998, another El Niño year, there were only two cases in the Northwest against eight in the Four Corners. If the Northwest is drier and the Southwest wetter in an El Niño, then the reverse may also be true. El Niño brings rain, and with it HPS, to the Four Corners and away from the northwest. So HPS is not a disease of the Four Corners states all of the time.

Even within the Four Corners, there are microclimates. In 1993, areas that had only recently experienced increased rainfall were the site of hantavirus cases, even though they were distant from the initial cluster in New Mexico. The first case in 1998 was high on a snow-covered mountain, one of the places where precipitation patterns are most consistent. It is likely that the moisture/mouse/morbidity model explains only some of the cases and that other factors are at work, which will be identified later.

"NEW" VIRUSES

Sin Nombre is one of a new class of viruses.

The viruses that kill large numbers of people were easy to spot. Smallpox, measles, and influenza were almost impossible to miss. Viruses that cause obvious disease in many people are also hard to miss: chicken pox, herpes, and the common cold. Also fairly obvious were the viruses, which, while rare, are killers: rabies and Ebola. Once seen, they are never forgotten.

A few eluded the net. Human herpesvirus 6, for example, has been identified only recently as the cause of erythema infectiosum, one of the "classic" childhood rashes. Most of the viruses that remain to be discovered, however, are relatively harmless, rare, or both, or so scientists believed.

Then came 1993 and a new virus, killing over half of its victims within days. It had been missed because it was a relatively minor cause of something similar to a common condition, adult respiratory distress syndrome, which kills between 50,000 and 150,000 Americans each year. So it was quite easy to overlook something that kills, on average, about 40 of them each year.

Are there any more out there? Yes, and they are probably doing the same kind of thing: killing a small number of people who are mistaken for part of a larger problem, such as heart disease, senility, or cancers. They may never account for the millions killed by smallpox, measles, or influenza, but they are killers all the same.

Whitewater Arroyo virus has been identified recently in the United States. It is a member of the family Arenaviridae, a relative of killers such as Lassa fever in Africa or Junin and Machupo in South America, but it belongs to a different branch of the family. So far, it seems to be harmless. Of course, it is not clear why if South American arenaviruses are killers, a new virus to the north should be harmless.

However, there are killers out there, some still unknown and some only recently discovered.

GENESIS OF A KILLER

Where did Sin Nombre come from? All the evidence suggests that hantaviruses have been evolving with their rodent hosts for a very long time, maybe even as long as those hosts have existed.

Could the virus have changed suddenly before the 1993 outbreak? After all, there was a huge El Niño event in 1982 and the virus was not discovered then. But review of the 1982 data failed to find any evidence of HPS-like disease. So why no HPS?

The first possibility is that the virus itself has changed.

SHIFTING AND DRIFTING

Hantaviruses, like all members of the virus family Bunyaviridae, keep their genes in three pieces ("segments") of RNA. Influenza A virus has eight RNA segments containing its genes. Swapping of genes is much easier when those genes are in multiple pieces—no cutting or no joining. With influenza, mixing of genes from strains infecting humans with those from strains infecting birds is thought to be the key to the appearance of the new "pandemic" strains that can dodge the immune system and sweep around the world. Mixed infections of pigs act as the "pressure cooker" for these new strains.

A wide variety of hantaviruses exist in similar animals, and it is known that they can infect animals other than their normal host. So mixing can happen, and swapping out one segment for a new one could change the virus dramatically.

It is an obvious explanation for the appearance of a new disease. It is a mechanism already known, with influenza, to produce significant human disease. It is obvious, but it did not happen with Sin Nombre.

The first clue was that antibodies from stored rodent and human specimens from many years before the 1993 outbreak seemed to recognize the "new" virus. However, that only covers part of the genes.

Then the actual genetic code was examined from these older samples. Again, the differences between them and the 1993 virus were not great. At first only part of the genetic code was known, but as more and more became available the evidence mounted that there had been few changes. Understanding of the meaning of the genetic code is not advanced enough to say that the small changes that were seen could not produce big effects. As mentioned earlier, a change of one letter of the genetic code changed one mild influenza virus into a certain killer.

However, the changes seemed to arise by the normal drift seen in virus genes as a result of random mutations. It just did not fit with the dramatic shifts expected if whole RNA segments were being exchanged.

Then, mixing of hantaviruses in cells grown in the laboratory was shown to produce gene swapping. Among Sin Nombre viruses taken from two different locations, mixing was common: 25 viruses of 294 produced in the experiment were mixtures of the two "parents." These were related too closely to produce big changes. When Sin Nombre and Black Creek Canal viruses were mixed, only 1 of 163 viruses was mixed.

In the words of Dr. Stuart Nichol, the leading expert on hantavirus molecular biology, "It was extremely difficult to get Sin Nombre–Black Creek Canal virus reassortants even out of experimental tissue culture mixed infections." The frequency of mixing was just too low to believe that it was happening in the wild at a level sufficient to explain the new outbreak of disease across such large areas.

That conclusion was supported by work with wild rodents. In a study in Texas, three different hantaviruses were circulating among four different types of rodent at the same location. Deer mice were carrying both Sin Nombre and El Moro Canyon viruses, yet no sign of genetic mixing was seen.

Dr. Brian Hjelle, a leading hantavirus expert, suggests that this is due to the strong adaptation of these viruses to their main host, such that any mixed virus will lose out in its "real" home and be selected against as a result. Evolution again.

HISTORY

The editor of the June 11, 1993, edition of *Morbidity and Mortality Weekly Report* in which HPS was first reported was Dr. Rick Goodman. In 1978, he had been out on his first case for the Epidemic Intelligence Service. It turned out not to be an outbreak of respiratory disease; it was a series of unconnected events, coincidences. However, one of the cases stuck in his mind: a young man with a sudden onset respiratory illness, whose lungs filled with fluid and who died despite the intensive care he was given. No cause was identified.

In 1993, Dr. Goodman pulled out the file, contacted the man's widow, and got permission to test tissue samples that had been stored at the time. The cause proved to have been the same hantavirus that was killing in the Four Corners.

Other clinicians recalled cases of unexplained ARDS in young, apparently healthy patients. For most of those, specimens were not available to test retroactively for hantavirus so the physicians could only speculate anecdotally, but speculate they did: that the disease was not new. A suspect case in 1959 has not been confirmed. The 1978 case remains the first fully authenticated case of HPS, but it is strong evidence that Sin Nombre was not "new" in 1993.

A BLOOM AND . . . SOMETHING ELSE

It was very clear that the 1993 outbreak in the Four Corners was linked to the massive increase in the number of rodents in the area: the "rodent bloom." The same effect was seen in Paraguay in 1995. The virus increases in frequency among rodents when there are more of them.

However, is one bloom enough?

There was a massive El Niño event in 1982, but no sign of HPS. There was a rodent bloom in 1991, almost as large as that in 1993, and yet intensive analysis of specimens from that time identified just one case of HPS. What was different?

Dr. Fred Koster of the University of New Mexico suggests that the bloom is the priming of outbreak. The winter after the bloom is the key event.

1998: "ALL THE CONDITIONS ARE IN PLACE"

In early 1998, health officials became concerned that climactic conditions resembled those of 1993 and that the Southwest might once again become an incubator for the still incurable disease. Warnings that "all the conditions are in place" for an outbreak of HPS were issued by the CDC and state health authorities. A wet spring had led to a large amount of vegetation in the Four Corners area. By now, rodent surveys were running across the Four Corners, run by a range of experts from institutions including the Sevilleta program and Colorado State University. Mouse numbers were rising in a way not seen since 1993. In some places, numbers were over three times higher than anything seen for the past 4 years. The percentage of mice showing antibody to hantavirus was also rising, approaching 1993 levels. The federal Occupational Safety and Health Administration cited a Gallup, New Mexico, hospital after one wing was found to be contaminated by mice.

The first 1998 HPS case was outside an area considered to be at high risk, which sparked fears that a greater number of people might face exposure. The conditions did indeed seem to be in place for another outbreak, but the alignment of causative factors did not occur.

First, crucially, the weather phenomenon that has come to be known as El Niño faltered. Later winter and early spring were wet in many areas, but not dramatically so. By late spring, the pattern had changed. The summer was dry, with precipitation dropping even lower than average in an area where "average" can be as little as 5 inches a year. The "monsoons," an ironic term in the high desert, were scant.

Second, another pattern had changed: human behavior. To begin with, nearly everyone had some baseline awareness of hantavirus, although it was not entirely factual. Author Tony Hillerman, whose mystery novels are set on the Navajo reservation, had mentioned the disease. The X-Files movie, a spin-off from the popular science-fiction series, had caught viewers' attention by mentioning alien visitation as a cause of HPS. The disease was also mentioned in *Playboy* magazine. Hantavirus did not come as a surprise this time.

Many residents were taking steps to control their exposure to rodents. Public health workers had begun early in the spring to alert people to the possible danger, and perhaps those lessons had taken hold.

Or had they?

FEAR AND FATALISM

Four Corners residents had been blessed with 5 years during which they could secure their homes and outbuildings against rodents, but 5 years was long enough for many to forget the fear they had felt in 1993, and so once again, many had adopted a rather cavalier attitude. Part of the culprit in such backsliding is surely the cyclical nature of hantavirus. Risk-taking behavior is not punished on a reliable basis, as most of the time the actual risk is small. By the time the incidence began to climb again, many residents had dropped the habit of taking precautions. Public health workers had to regain ground lost since the last outbreak before they could make real progress in averting the next one. They had to convince people that the risk, although small, was real. Because they were dealing with a culture (among both Indians and Anglos) that honored nature and an economy that depended on visitation, they had to be very careful with the psychological tools they chose to use.

Educational efforts had probably not been sufficiently effective that they alone could prevent an outbreak. Many of the residents who paid lip service to rodent control were somewhat fatalistic about their own risks. No one carried around a spray bottle of bleach solution and few people really disinfected every place that showed signs of rodent habitation or wore masks every time they entered a closed-up outbuilding. Both of the authors of this book were guilty of this. Colleagues of one of the authors delighted in making gifts of live mice trapped in other parts of the office. Far from being disinfected or isolated, they were quite lively and were contained only in cardboard boxes. Like many people, those co-workers had settled on a peaceful, if nervous, coexistence with *P. maniculatus.*

The lack of fear had a darker side as well.

PERENNIAL PREJUDICE

When news reports began circulating about the possibility of another outbreak, the opposition of the tourism-oriented business owners was apparent immediately. They protested that all the talk about HPS was ruining their business once again. Even though epidemiological studies had shown that non-Indians were at considerable risk, many Anglos insisted it was an Indian disease.

"It's only for Indians and people who live in filth," said the owner of one trading post during the spring of 1998 in a phone call complaining to a newspaper editor and canceling his advertising. When advised that the newspaper's writers believed they had a legitimate role in advising their readers of potential, and preventable, health risks, another businessman said that local subscribers should get that sort of news from the newspaper in the next town. (He did not, however, believe local shoppers should buy their Indian jewelry in the next town as well.) What would happen if businessmen in that next town felt the same way was not made clear.

"Put it in the paper when we have a case in Colorado," another anonymous complainant suggested. "What happens on the res (reservation) doesn't have anything to do with us."

The next case *was* in Colorado, and the victim was an Anglo woman, well-educated, professional, and financially secure.

In 1998, though, business did not suffer nearly as much as it had in 1993. A chamber of commerce spokesperson from Farmington, New Mexico—the town with the deserted Main

Street in 1993—reported only two calls inquiring about hanta-virus during the entire summer. It was no longer new and no longer very interesting.

REAL-LIFE RISK FACTORS

Most people who didn't want to hear about the disease didn't believe that they were at risk. They lived in houses, not trailers, they'd point out. They would insist that they didn't have mice (although Charles Calisher, an expert in the field, has said he could find mice in nearly anyone's house).

Most southwesterners, even those who live in the middle of town, have a decidedly rural life-style. Many heat their homes with wood, many have gardens, and many Four Corners residents live in rural areas, sharing an ecosystem with deer mice and a host of other animals.

Whether or not they are willing to admit it, those people are at some risk. Those who have woodpiles very likely have mice nesting there. Those who have sheds or barns undoubtedly have mice as well. Mice, not poverty or ethnic origin, are the risk. Americans live in a free country; they can believe what they choose. They can believe that they are immune because they're not Native American and they can believe that their "superior" standard of living will protect them.

And they can die of ignorance. Sometimes, they do.

IGNORANCE KILLS; EDUCATION SAVES

Certainly the number of cases was higher in 1993. In the Four Corners states, the number was sufficiently higher that simple statistical testing showed that it was unlikely to have happened by random chance. Dr. Brian Hjelle of the University of New Mexico believes that 1998 was an outbreak year, but public health education and a "real fear" of rodents were what prevented the number of cases from being far higher.

There are alternative explanations for why the 1998 outbreak did not happen at the level of 1993.

WINTER KILLS

When rodent numbers are low, rodents are found mainly in "refugia," which are relatively small areas with enough food and shelter to support larger numbers of rodents. This is well known, and refugia have been identified for some species. There appears to be a mouse refugia high up in the northwestern corner of the Sevilleta site south of Albuquerque, for example. Outside these refugia, rodent numbers may be very low indeed.

Rodents are short lived, perhaps no more than 6 months for an average deer mouse in the wild. Hantavirus needs to keep infecting new rodents if it is to remain in the rodent population. If the rodent hosts are widely scattered, it may not be able to do so. When rodent numbers are low, hantaviruses may be eliminated from the rodent population outside the refugia. Again, this is known to happen.

When a bloom occurs, both rodents and virus need to spread out from the refugia. As they spread, a relatively small number of humans may be exposed, causing scattered cases of the disease.

If a rodent bloom is followed by a cold, harsh winter, rodent numbers will fall dramatically. The next year, rodents and viruses will be back in the refugia. However, if the winter is warm, rodents will survive. If a crop such as piñon nuts is plentiful, there will be food through the winter.

What will the rodents be doing all winter? Becoming infected. Winter is cold. Rodents are small. They need to huddle, inside burrows or other shelter. The big, male rodents that carry hantavirus will fight. In close-living conditions, crowded as a result of the bloom, the number of rodents carrying hantavirus could increase dramatically.

If the bloom and the warm, well-fed winter are followed by a wet, fertile spring, the extra food can allow an extra breeding cycle for the rodents, so there are even more mice the next year and now they are infected. The virus is out of the refugia.

1998 could have been an outbreak year prevented by public education or it could have been the scattered cases around the refugia—the priming.

The need for a bloom, a fertile crop in the fall, a warm winter, and a wet spring could explain why an outbreak like 1993 is unusual. The more factors required to converge, the less frequent will be such occurrences.

The year 1998 saw a rodent bloom, not all through the year, but numbers were up. The *Albuquerque Journal* of October 3, 1998, carried a story about a bumper crop of piñon nuts in some parts of New Mexico. In other areas, however, crop was less plentiful; in southwestern Colorado it was nearly nonexistent.

At the time of this writing, it is not known whether the winter of 1998–1999 will be warm—it began early and cold—or whether the spring of 1999 will be wet. However, coming after a rodent bloom and a fertile piñon crop, 1999 is a time with a clear and identifiable risk, if this model is true.

Maybe winter conditions will avert the spread of the virus. Maybe the factors will not all fall into place this year, or next. Eventually, they will, and hantavirus infection of humans will emerge.

Maybe 1998 was the year of the outbreak, stopped by steel wool and Lysol. But maybe it wasn't. Time will give us the answer to this, as to so many questions. It may not be the answer that we want.

APPENDIX A
Centers for Disease Control Guidelines on Prevention of HPS

TIPS FOR PREVENTING HPS

Prevention Indoors and Outdoors

Indoors

• Keep a clean home, especially the kitchen (wash dishes, clean counters and floor, and keep food covered in rodent-proof containers).

• Keep a tight-fitting lid on garbage and discard uneaten pet food at the end of the day.

• Set and keep spring-loaded rodent traps. Set traps near baseboards as rodents tend to run along walls and tight spaces rather than out in the open.

• Set EPA-approved rodenticide with bait under plywood or plastic shelter along baseboards. These are sometimes known as "covered bait stations." Remember to follow product use instructions carefully, as rodenticides are also poisonous to pets and people.

- If bubonic plague is a problem in your area, spray flea killer or spread flea powder in the area before setting traps. This is important. If you control rodents but do not control fleas as well, you may increase the risk of infection with bubonic plague, as fleas will leave rodents once the rodents die and will seek out other food sources, including humans.

- Seal all entry holes ¼ inch wide or wider with steel wool, cement, wire screening, or other patching materials, inside and out.

Outdoors

- Clear brush, grass, and junk from around house foundations to eliminate a source of nesting materials.

- Use metal flashing around the base of wooden, earthen, or adobe homes to provide a strong metal barrier. Install so that the flashing reaches 12 inches above the ground and 6 inches down into the ground.

- Elevate hay, woodpiles, and garbage cans to eliminate possible nesting sites. If possible, locate them 100 feet or more from your house.

- Trap rodents outside, too. Poisons or rodenticides may be used as well, but be sure to keep them out of the reach of children or pets.

- Encourage natural predators such as nonpoisonous snakes, owls, and hawks.

- Remember, totally getting rid of all rodents isn't feasible, but with ongoing effort you can keep the population very low.

How Do I Clean Up a Rodent-Infested Area?

Clean Up Infested Areas, Using Safety Precautions:
- Put on latex rubber gloves before cleaning up.

- Don't stir up dust by sweeping or vacuuming up droppings, urine, or nesting materials.

- Instead, wet contaminated areas thoroughly with detergent or liquid to deactivate the virus. Most general-purpose disinfectants and household detergents are effective. However, a hypochlorite solution prepared by mixing 1.5 cups of household bleach in 1 gallon of water may be used in place of commercial disinfectant. When using the chlorine solution, avoid spilling the mixture on clothing or other items that may be damaged.

- Once everything is wet, take up contaminated materials with a damp towel and then mop or sponge the area with disinfectant.

- Spray dead rodents with disinfectant, double bag along with all cleaning materials, and bury, burn, or throw out in appropriate waste disposal system. If burning or burying isn't feasible, contact your local or state health department about other disposal methods.

- Finally, disinfect gloves *before taking them off* with disinfectant or soap and water. After taking off the clean gloves, wash hands thoroughly with soap and warm water.

When going into cabins or outbuildings (or work areas) that have been closed for awhile, open them up and air out before cleaning.

What If My House or Workplace is Infested Heavily with Rodents?

You should get help from a professional exterminator if you see many droppings or rodents, as you may have a bad infestation problem, or you can contact your local health authorities for advice. CDC has recommendations for how heavy infestations may be handled most safely.

What If I Work Around Rodents Frequently? What Should I Do?

You may wish to read the specific CDC recommendations for workers in affected areas who are exposed regularly to rodents.

Why All the Fuss about Spraying Disinfectant, Washing Traps with Bleach, and Such?

These viruses are surrounded by a lipid (fatty) envelope so they are somewhat fragile. The lipid envelope can be destroyed and the virus killed by fat solvents such as alcohol, ordinary disinfectants, and household bleach. That is why one of the most important ways to prevent transmitting the disease is to carefully wet down dead rodents and areas where rodents have been with disinfectant and/or bleach. When you do this, you are killing the virus itself and reducing the chance that the virus will get into the air.

Summing Up

How to Prevent HPS

- Make your home, workplace, and vacation home unattractive to them
- Clean up infested areas using safety precautions
- Wet down infested areas with bleach/disinfectant to kill the virus before it aerosolizes
- in other words: AIR OUT, SEAL UP, TRAP UP, AND CLEAN UP

SPECIAL PRECAUTIONS FOR HOMES OF PERSONS WITH CONFIRMED HANTAVIRUS INFECTION OR BUILDINGS WITH HEAVY RODENT INFESTATIONS

Special precautions should be used for cleaning homes or buildings with heavy rodent infestations in areas where HPS has been reported. If you are attempting to deal with such an infestation, it is recommended that you contact the responsible local, state, or federal public health agency for guidance.

Special precautions may also apply to vacant dwellings that have attracted numbers of rodents while unoccupied and to dwellings and other structures that have been occupied by persons with confirmed hantavirus infection.

Workers who are either hired specifically to perform the cleanup or asked to do so as part of their work activities should receive a thorough orientation from the responsible health agency about hantavirus transmission and should be trained to perform the required activities safely.

Precautions to Be Used

• A baseline serum sample, preferably drawn at the time these prevention activities are initiated, should be available for all persons conducting the cleanup of homes or buildings with heavy rodent infestation. The serum sample should be stored at $-20°C$.

• Persons involved in the cleanup should wear coveralls (disposable, if possible), rubber boots or disposable shoe covers, rubber or plastic gloves, protective goggles, and an appropriate respiratory protection device, such as a half-mask air-purifying (or negative-pressure) respirator with a high-efficiency particulate air (HEPA) filter or a powered air-purifying respirator (PAPR) with HEPA filters. Respirators (including positive-pressure types) are not considered protective if facial hair interferes with the face seal, as proper fit cannot be assured. Respirator practices should follow a comprehensive user program and be supervised by a knowledgeable person.

• Personal protective gear should be decontaminated upon removal at the end of the day. If the coveralls are not disposable, they should be laundered on site. If no laundry facilities are available, the coveralls should be immersed in liquid disinfectant until they can be washed.

• All potentially infective waste material (including respirator filters) from cleanup operations that cannot be burned or deep buried on site should be double bagged in appropriate plastic bags. The bagged material should then be labeled as infectious (if it is to be transported) and disposed of in accordance with local requirements for infectious waste.

• Workers who develop symptoms suggestive of HPS within 45 days of the last potential exposure should seek medical attention immediately. The physician should contact local health authorities promptly if hantavirus-associated illness is suspected. A blood sample should be obtained and forwarded with the baseline serum through the state health department to CDC for hantavirus antibody testing.

PRECAUTIONS FOR WORKERS IN AFFECTED AREAS WHO ARE REGULARLY EXPOSED TO RODENTS

Persons who frequently handle or are exposed to rodents (e.g., mammalogists, pest control workers) in the affected area are probably at higher risk for hantavirus infection than the general public because of their frequency of exposure. Therefore, enhanced precautions are warranted to protect them against hantavirus infection.

Precautions to Be Used

• A baseline serum sample, preferably drawn at the time of employment, should be available for all persons whose occupations involve frequent rodent contact. The serum sample should be stored at $-20°C$.

• Workers in potentially high-risk settings should be informed about the symptoms of the disease and be given detailed guidance on prevention measures.

• Workers who develop a febrile or respiratory illness within 45 days of the last potential exposure should seek medical attention immediately and inform the attending physician of the potential occupational risk of hantavirus infection. The physician should contact local health authorities promptly if hantavirus-associated illness is suspected. A blood sample should be obtained and forwarded with the baseline serum through the state health department to CDC for hantavirus antibody testing.

• Workers should wear a half-face air-purifying (or negative-pressure) respirator or PAPR equipped with HEPA filters when removing rodents from traps or handling rodents in the affected area. Respirators (including positive-pressure types) are not considered protective if facial hair interferes with the face seal, as proper fit cannot be assured. Respirator-use practices should be in accord with a comprehensive user program and should be supervised by a knowledgeable person.

• Workers should wear rubber or plastic gloves when handling rodents or handling traps containing rodents. Gloves should be washed and disinfected before removing them, as described earlier.

• Traps contaminated by rodent urine or feces or in which a rodent was captured should be disinfected with a commercial disinfectant or bleach solution. Dispose of dead rodents as described earlier.

- Persons removing organs or obtaining blood from rodents in affected areas should contact the Special Pathogens Branch, Division of Viral and Rickettsial Diseases, National Center for Infectious Diseases, Centers for Disease Control and Prevention [telephone (404) 639-1115] for detailed safety precautions.

PRECAUTIONS FOR OTHER OCCUPATIONAL GROUPS WHO HAVE POTENTIAL RODENT CONTACT

Insufficient information is available at this time to allow general recommendations regarding risks or precautions for persons in affected areas who work in occupations with unpredictable or incidental contact with rodents or their habitations. Examples of such occupations include telephone installers, maintenance workers, plumbers, electricians, and certain construction workers. Workers in these jobs may have to enter various buildings, crawl spaces, or other sites that may be rodent infested. Recommendations for such circumstances must be made on a case-by-case basis after the specific working environment has been assessed and state or local health departments have been consulted.

HANTAVIRUS HOTLINE

You may telephone CDC to obtain information on the hantavirus pulmonary syndrome. The number is 1-800-532-9929. Please note that information offered is at the same level, or less detailed, than that found on the CDC website at http://www.cdc.gov/ncidod/diseases/hanta/hps/index.htm

APPENDIX B
Sources of Further Information

The Coming Plague

Laurie Garrett, Penguin Books, 1994

ISBN 0140250913

An excellent and wide-ranging account of many "new" or emerging diseases. Written in a readable and informed style, it covers everything from malaria to hantavirus via toxic shock syndrome and AIDS. It is highly detailed, but because of its broad coverage, most topics are restricted to a chapter or less. AIDS is an exception. Chapter 15 covers the 1993 outbreak of Sin Nombre hantavirus.

Virus Hunter: Thirty Years of Battling Hot Viruses Around the World

C. J. Peters and Mark Olshaker, Anchor Books, 1997

ISBN 0385485581

An autobiographical account from one of the world's most renowned "virus hunters." C. J. Peters' life, from west Texas oil-town boyhood to the end of the 1993 Sin Nombre virus outbreak. Most of it spent in the military, with inside information on many aspects of that work, including biological weapons programs. Very readable, containing many of the "real" details that puts even advanced science on a human scale.

Virus X: Tracking the New Killer Plagues

Frank Ryan, Back Bay Books, 1997
ISBN 0316763063

A very personal view of the subject from a British virologist. The main focus of the book is the methods by which "new" and emerging viruses appear and plagues develop. The 1993 hantavirus outbreak occupies six chapters, but again coverage stops with the "end" of that outbreak. The book contains many details and idiosyncratic theories, some of them discussed in the text of this book.

The Hot Zone

Richard Preston, Anchor Books, 1995
ISBN 0385479565

Almost the defining "popular" account of virus hunting. An account of the discovery of Ebola virus in an animal facility a few miles from Washington D.C. in 1989. Although this version of the virus was found to be (apparently) harmless to humans, some types of Ebola kill up to 90% of those infected. The description of the fear and the reaction to the virus is compelling.

The Encyclopedia of Mammals

David W. MacDonald, Facts on File Publications, 1995
ISBN 0871968711

A huge information resource filled with pictures and information on everything from deer mice to lions.

USA Today

Steve Sternberg, July 2nd and July 6th 1998

A series of articles on hantavirus, concentrating on the circumstances surrounding the index cases in 1993. Very readable and highly detailed.

For More Detail

Hantavirus infection

Gregory J. Mertz, Brian L. Hjelle, and Ralph T. Bryan.
Advances in Internal Medicine, **volume 42, pages 369–421.**
Mosby-Year Book, Inc. 1997.

A professional review of the subject, but very, very readable, up to date and wide ranging.

Molecular Virology

David R. Harper, Bios Scientific Publishers/Springer.
200 pages. 1998.
ISBN 1859962467

Much more detail on how viruses actually work. Written for a college audience, but may be helpful to the curious.

The Real Thing

The most important resource used when this book was being written was the internet. It would have been impossible to write in its current form without this instant source of up-to-date information. Because of the "hypertext" nature of the internet, most of the following pages are connected by "links" from individual pages to others on the list. The following websites were most used by the authors.

http://www.cdc.gov/ncidod/diseases/hanta/hps/index.htm
Centers for Disease Control Hantavirus information page
A huge resource of information on all aspects of hantavirus disease in the United States including latest case numbers, with many links to related information sources. Well written and (generally) up to date with information at general and technical levels.

http://thor.unm.edu/Hanta/Website1.htm#recog
University of New Mexico Hantavirus Reference Laboratory information pages
A wide range of information from a very active group working on clinical and research aspects of hantavirus pulmonary syndrome, including details of diagnosis and testing of samples from patients as well as the ongoing ribavirin trial.

http://www.cdphe.state.co.us/hanta/hanta.html
The Colorado Department of Public Health and Environment maintains a hantavirus web page with information for physicians as well as answers to the most commonly asked questions about the disease.

http://www.healthnet.org/programs/promed.html#archives
ProMED Mail
The Program for Monitoring Emerging Diseases.
A full archive of the daily email "heads up" service used by a mixture of leading experts and interested amateurs worldwide. The questions and answers in this heady brew range from abstruse technical jargon to serious sarcasm. It is always informative and provides one of the finest guides to health issues across the world. The (free) email subscription service can be accessed from this site.

http://www.reutershealth.com
Reuters health news service.
The "popular" digest (Health eLine) is free, other services require subscription.

http://www.cdc.gov/ncidod/eid/index.htm
Emerging Infectious Diseases online
A professional journal on the topic published by the National Center for Infectious Diseases that contains excellent and highly readable technical reviews.

http://www.outbreak.org/cgi-unreg/dynaserve.exe/index.html
Outbreak
An on-line information service addressing emerging diseases, with details of many of the current and recent problems around the world.

http://www.cdc.gov/epo/mmwr/mmwr.html
Morbidity and Mortality Weekly Report
Downloadable version of the Centers for Disease Control's own "house journal." A very uncatchy name and more a collection of statistics than something to read, but very much "the horse's mouth" for information on disease within the United States.

http://sevilleta.unm.edu
Sevilleta long-term ecological research program website
Information on all aspects of the work of the program, including the rodent surveys, which form a major element of understanding hantavirus disease in the United States.

http://www.elnino.noaa.gov/
National Oceanic and Atmospheric Administration El Niño information page
A rich source of information on all aspects of the El Niño event presented in a readable and very informative way.

http://www.minsal.cl/epidemiologia/hantas/index.htm
Chilean Ministry of Health Information website
Up-to-date information on hantavirus disease in Chile. In Spanish, but with many tables that need no translation. The translation service at http://babelfish.altavista.com/cgi-bin/translate? can provide rough translations of any text.

http://www.healthig.com/English/hantav1.html
Argentinian news service (Health I.G. Consultora Periodística) hantavirus information website
Contains informative and highly detailed accounts of outbreaks of hantavirus disease in Argentina, including a great deal of hard to find information, especially about the El Bolson outbreak. More up-to-date information is also available in Spanish. Again, the automated translation service at http://babelfish.altavista.com/cgi-bin/translate? can provide approximate translations.

http://www.tulane.edu/~dmsander/garryfavwebindex.html
"All the Virology on the World-wide Web"
The ultimate resource for all things relating to viruses. It is possible to get almost any information on viruses within a few clicks from this page.

General Four Corners information
http://www.fourcorners.com

Official websites for the Four Corners states
http://www.state.az.us
http://www.state.co.us
http://www.state.nm.us
http://www.state.ut.us

Attractions mentioned in the book
Arizona
http://hanksville.phast.umass.edu/defs/monval/monval.html
Monument Valley Navajo Tribal Park
http://www.nps.gov/cach/
Canyon de Chelly National Monument

Colorado
http://www.nps.gov/meve/
Mesa Verde National Park

Utah
http://www.nps.gov/cany/
Canyonlands National Park
http://moab-utah.com/rack/dhpsp.html
Dead Horse Point State Park

New Mexico
http://www.nps.gov/chcu/
Chaco Culture National Historical Park
http://www.nps.gov/peco/
Pecos National Historical Park

APPENDIX C
Abbreviations

A	Adenosine, a subunit of DNA (properly, deoxyadenine) or RNA
AIDS	Acquired immune deficiency syndrome
ARDS	Adult respiratory distress syndrome
C	Cytidine, a subunit of DNA (properly, deoxycytosine) or RNA
CDC	Centers for Disease Control and Prevention, the main U.S. disease monitoring organization, based in Atlanta, Georgia.
DNA	Deoxyribonucleic acid, the material of the genes
ECMO	Extracorporeal membrane oxygenation
G	Guanosine, a subunit of DNA (properly, deoxyguanine) or RNA
H or HA	Hemagglutinin, an outer protein of influenza virus
HEPA	High efficiency particulate air (filter)
HFRS	Hemorrhagic fever with renal syndrome, the Eurasian hantavirus disease
HIV	Human immunodeficiency virus, the cause of AIDS

HLA	Human leukocyte antigen, marker proteins on the surfaces of white blood cells that are involved with the immune response
HPS	Hantavirus pulmonary syndrome
KGB	Komitet Gosurdarstvennoy Besopasnasti, translated as the "Committee for State Security"
LTER	Long term ecological research
MMWR	Morbidity and Mortality Weekly Report, the "house journal" of the CDC
N or NA	Neuraminidase, an outer protein of influenza virus
NE	Nephropathia epidemica, the milder European form of HFRS
NIH	National Institutes of Health
PAPR	Powered air-purifying respirator
PCR	Polymerase chain reaction, a biochemical technique to produce huge numbers of copies of a small segment of a gene
RNA	Ribonucleic acid, a cellular messenger molecule and the genetic material of most viruses
SV	Simian virus
T	Thymidine, a subunit of DNA (properly, deoxythymidine)
U	Uridine, a subunit of RNA, the equivalent of thymidine in DNA
UN	United Nations
UNM	University of New Mexico
US	United States
USAMRIID	United States Army Medical Research Institute of Infectious Disease, based at Fort Detrick, Maryland

INDEX

Acquired immunodeficiency
    syndrome (AIDS), 142,
    179–180; *see also* Human
    immunodeficiency virus
Adult respiratory distress
    syndrome (ARDS), 8, 192, 200
    annual deaths from, 238
    as suspect HPS cases, 241
Age
    of HFRS patients, 107
    of HPS patients, 234
    in Argentina, 192
Albuquerque Journal, 14, 247
Alexander, Harold (Lord), 102
Altitude, mouse populations and
    infection levels, 72–73
American meadow vole (*Microtus
    pennsylvanicus*), 126
Amplification, viral, 177
    by population movement, 179
    by poverty, 180
Andes virus, 193–194, 209, 232

transmission of, 202
Anglos, attitudes on and cases of
    HPV among, 81, 89, 234, 244
Anthrax, 155–156
Antibodies
    to Ebola in Zaire, 181
    to hantavirus, and disease
      incidence, 203
    to Sin Nombre virus
      and disease prevalence,
      204–205
      in Four Corners rodents,
      68–69
    testing for, 210
Antigenic drift, 165
Antigenic shift
    hantavirus, 239
    influenza virus, 169
Antiviral drugs, 213, 220; *see also*
    Ribavirin
Apoptosis, 141
Arboviruses, 153

Arenaviridae, 238
Argentina, hantavirus disease in,
    189–192, 196
Arthropod-borne viruses, 153
Asian striped field mouse
    (*Apodemus agrarius*), 31
    identification as viral source,
    109
Athabascan migrations, 207
Autoimmune disease, 213
Aztec nation, 149–150

Baculoviruses, in biological
    control, 159–160
Bahe, Merrill, 6–7, 12, 34, 203
Balkans, 121
Baltimore rat virus, 115
Bandicoot rat (*Bandicota indica*),
    123
Bank vole (*Clethrionomys glareolus*),
    72, 119
Bashkortostan (Russia), 122
Bayou virus, 184–185, 188, 190
Belgium, HFRS in, 120
Berkelman, Ruth, 22
Biological control, 158
Black Creek Canal hantavirus, 185,
    187
    genetic mixing with Sin
        Nombre, 240
Black rat (*Rattus rattus*), 113
Bloodland Lake hantavirus,
    187
Bosnia, HFRS deaths in, 121
Bouquet, Henry, 17, 150
Brazil, hantavirus disease in,
    188–189
Brieman, Rob, 22

Brown rat (*Rattus norvegicus*), 31,
    113
Brush mouse (*Peromyscus boylii*), 65
Bunyaviridae, 71, 111
    segmented genome of, 239
Butler, Jay, 22

Cactus mouse (*Peromyscus eremicus*),
    65
Caliciviridae, 157
Calisher, Charles, 45, 111, 196, 245
Campbell, Thomas B., 63
Canada
    gender and HPV, 235
    Sin Nombre virus in, 197
Cañon del Muerto, 96
Canyon de Chelly, 96
Canyonlands National Park, 65
Carbonyl chloride, 10
Cardiopulmonary support, with
    ECMO, 230
Carriman, Flora, 190
Centers for Disease Control, 21, 35
    field investigations of, 23
    HPS clinical case definition,
        200
    laboratory criteria for HPS
        diagnosis, 201
    specimen analysis at, 28–31
    treatment protocols of, 87
    viral research by, 92–93
Chaco Canyon, 48
Cheek, Jim, 7, 14
Chicken pox, 146, 217
Childs, Jamie, 128
Chile, hantavirus disease in,
    193–194, 196
    gender as factor, 235

China, Hantaan infection in, 105
mortality and risk factors, 106
Circe retrovirus, 175
Civil War, 103, 115
Climate, of Four Corners region, 20
Colilargo mouse, 189, 190, 222
Containment levels, for infectious agents, 28
Cornaglia, Susan, 191
Cortéz, Hernán, 149
Cortez (Colorado), tourism in, 84
Cortizo de Nassif, Esther, 190
Cotton rat (*Sigmodon hispidus*), 185, 187
Croatia, 121

Deer mouse (*Peromyscus maniculatus*), 65, 68, 149, 245
breeding patterns, 61–62
in Canada, 197
control efforts, 80–81
hantavirus antibodies, 69
identification as virus carrier, 48
Deoxyribonucleic acid (DNA), 32, 132–133, 137
in retroviruses, 171–172
in vaccinea, 218
Dobrava virus, 121
"Drowning sickness," 46
Drug resistance, development of, 166–167

Ebola virus, 142, 146
passive immunization, 217
poverty as amplifier of, 180–181
Zaire versus Reston strains, 149

ECMO, *see* Extracorporeal membrane oxygenation
Education efforts, 38–39, 226–227
El Bolson (Argentina), hantavirus disease in, 190–192
El Moro Canyon hantavirus, 187, 188, 190, 240
El Niño, 49, 228
and HPS incidence, 236–237, 241
link with rodent population, 62, 236
and Rift Valley fever, 154
water temperature and energy effects, 50–51
weather effects, 51–52
El Niño/southern oscillation (ENSO), 52
Epidemic benign nephropathy, 118
Epidemic hemorrhagic fever, 103
Erythema infectiosum, 237
Europe; *see also specific country*
HFRS laboratory outbreaks, 114
European common vole (*Microtus arvalis*), 123
Evolution
hantaviruses and rodents, in North America, 125
mutation as driving force, 164
Extracorporeal membrane oxygenation (ECMO), 230

Fort Pitt, 17
Four Corners region, 2
agency jurisdiction in, 22–23
altitude, 73
ancestral Puebloans, 56–57

Four Corners region *(continued)*
  conditions for outbreak in 1998,
    242–243
  description of, 2–4
  media outlets of, 66–67
  mice in, 36, 38
  population, 42
    and Sin Nombre antibody
      prevalence, 205
  risk taking behavior in, 243–244
  rodent surveys
    1993, 68
    1998, 242
  topography, 137
  tourism industry and media
    attention, 82–84
  weather, 53–56

Gabriel, Kathryn, 47
Gadjusek, Carleton, 117, 125–126
Gender, as factor in hantavirus
    infection, 107, 235
Gene swapping, in influenza, 168
  effects of, 164–165
Gene therapy, 160–161
Genetic engineering, limits of, 157
Geneva Protocol of 1925, 10
Genomes, segmented, in viruses,
    167, 171, 239
Goodman, Rick, 240, 241
Gran Chaco (Paraguay), 194–195
Greece, 122

Hantaan virus, 31
  first report of, 143
  infection in mouse host, 70, 109
  sensitivity to ribavirin, 85–86

transmission, 107, 202
  vaccine for, 128, 219
Hantavirus-associated adult
    respiratory distress syndrome,
    38; *see also* Hantavirus
    pulmonary syndrome
Hantaviruses
  antibody presence and disease
    incidence, 203–204
  in Argentina, 189–192
  in Brazil, 188–189
  characteristics of genus, 111
  in Chile, 193–194
  in Europe, 117–124
  Four Corners, *see* Sin Nombre
    virus
  host-based subdivisions of, 124
  incubation period, 202
  known types, 34
  in Paraguay, 194–195
  research funding, 129, 231–232
  seasonality of, 76–77, 223
  vaccines against, 218–219
Hantavirus infection
  in American rodent hosts,
    72–73
  in Asian rodent hosts, 70–71
  in Europe, 117; *see also* Puumala
    virus
    rodent hosts, 71–72
  historical records, in Asia,
    104–105
  prejudice against victims of, 90
  renal, recovery from, 103
Hantavirus pulmonary syndrome
    (HPS), 14
  CDC clinical definition,
    199–200
  as classic zoonosis, 151–152

clustering of, 206
early suspect cases, 241
and HLA type, 207
immune response as causation,
    210–213
laboratory criteria, 201
naming of, 93–94
number of new cases, 215
pattern of illness, 39–40
recovery from, 89, 231
risk from single exposure,
    203–205
symptoms, 38, 211
treatment protocols, 86–87,
    229–231
Hantavirus Study Site, 74–75
Health agencies, public education
    efforts by, 38–39
Hemagglutinin, 164, 168
Hemorrhagic fever with renal
    syndrome (HFRS), 31, 105
age and gender variations in, 107
laboratory outbreaks, 114
misdiagnosis of, 116
Hemorrhagic kidney disease, 85
Hepatitis, 178
immune response in, 210
Herpesviridae, 178
Herpesvirus 6, 178, 237
HFRS, *see* Hemorrhagic fever with
    renal syndrome
High desert
description of, 2
ecology of, 54
    long-term ecological research
        programs, 63
    rodent adaptation to, 49
precipitation, 54–56
Hillerman, Tony, 242

HIV, *see* Human
    immunodeficiency virus
Hjelle, Brian, 124, 240, 245
Hong Kong flu
    H3N2 (1968), 168
    H5N1 (1997), 170
Hopi, 15
    resistance to hantavirus among,
        208
House mouse (*Mus musculus*), 126
Ho Wang Lee, 109, 115, 126
Hoyle, Fred, 20
HPS, *see* Hantavirus pulmonary
    syndrome
Human immunodeficiency virus
    (HIV), 172
    amplification of, 179–180
    as biowarfare agent, 156
    drug resistance in, 166
    as zoonosis, 152
Human leukocyte antigen (HLA),
    206
    HLA-B*35, 207, 208, 213
Humans
    as end-stage host, 209–210
    in hantavirus life, 69–70
Humboldt current, 50

Immune response, 141, 173
    role of human leukocyte
        antigen, 206–207
    in viral disease, 210–213
Immunization; *see also* Vaccines
    passive, 217
Indian Health Service, 13, 44
    harm-reduction efforts, 79, 81
Infectious agents, containment
    level classification, 28

Influenza
   Fort Dix outbreak (1976),
      169–170
   Hong Kong
      H3N2 (1968), 168
      H5N1 (1997), 170
   pandemic, 167–171
   "Spanish" (1918–1920), 10, 25
   mortality from, 169
Influenza virus, surface proteins,
   164
   antigenic shift, 168–169
   mutations of, 165
Ingersoll, Robert, 179
Integrins, 20
Isla Vista hantavirus, 187
Ivanofsky, Dimitri, 129

Jahrling, Peter, 128
Japan, virus research, 108
Juquitiba virus, 188

Khabarovsk virus, 123
Kidney disease, hemorrhagic, 85
Kidneys; see also Hemorrhagic fever
   with renal syndrome
   effects of Korean hemorrhagic
      fever, 103
Kinshasa Highway, 179
Korean hemorrhagic fever, 103
   gender as factor, 235
   mortality from, 104
Korean vole (Eothenomys regulus),
   120
Korean War, 100–102
   spread of Hantaan infection
      following, 105–106

Koster, Fred, 195, 209, 230, 241
Ksiazek, Thomas G., 128

Laguna Negra hantavirus, 194
   antibody to, among Indians, 203
Lake Powell, 3
Landsat survey satellites, 228
La Niña, 52–53
Lassa fever, 30, 171
Laurasia, 125
Legionnaire's disease, 16
Lemmings, 119
   population cycles, 71–72
   Siberian (Lemmus sibericus), 123
Leukocytes, 211
Life
   basic machinery of, 132–133
   early theories of origins,
      133–134
Long-tailed pygmy rice rat
      (Oligoryzomys longicaudatus),
      189, 190
Long-term ecological research
      programs (LTER), 63
"Long Walk," 57
Los Alamos (New Mexico), 18
Los Angeles, 115
LTER, see Long-term ecological
      research programs
Lungs; see also Hantavirus
      pulmonary syndrome (HPS)
   damage from Puumala
      infection, 118

Manchuria, 108
   hantavirus disease in, 105
Manhatten Project, 18

Marburg virus, 181
Martín, Roberto, 191
McFeeley, Patty, 6, 10
Meadow vole (*Microtus arvalis*), 31
Measles, 177
Media coverage
  of El Bolson outbreak, 192
  of Four Corners outbreak, 37,
    65–67
  criticism of, 222
Mennonites, in Paraguay, HPS
    incidence among, 195
Mice
  Asian striped field (*Apodemus
    agrarius*), 31, 70, 109
  brush (*Peromyscus boylii*), 65
    hantavirus antibodies, 69
  cactus (*Peromyscus eremicus*), 65
  deer (*Peromyscus maniculatus*),
    48, 61–62, 65, 68, 69,
    80–81, 149, 197, 245
  house (*Mus musculus*), 126
  piñon (*Peromyscus truei*), 48, 65,
    69
  vesper (*Calomys laucha*), 194
  western harvest (*Reithrodontomys
    megalotis*), 187
  white-footed (*Peromyscus
    leucopus*), 65, 186, 197
  yellow-necked field (*Apodemus
    flavicollis*), 121
Microtinae, 124
Miller, Stanley, 136
Mites, Hantaan virus in, 71
MMWR, *see Morbidity and Mortality
    Weekly Report*
Monoclonal antibodies, 32
Monongahela virus, 187
Moose, Puumala antibody in, 119

*Morbidity and Mortality Weekly
    Report*, 35, 36, 240
  on rodent survey results, 48
Moreno de Gozólez, Adriana, 191
Mormon pioneers, 57–58
Mortality rate
  Andes HPS, 193
  Dorbrava hantavirus, 121
  Ebola virus, 149
  Korean hemorrhagic fever, 104
    in China, 106
    recent, 105
  Rift Valley fever, 154
  Sin Nombre HPS, 92
    in Canada, 197
    improvements in, 229
Mosquitos, in transmission of Rift
    Valley fever, 154
Mouse kachinas, 45
Muju virus, 123
Muleshoe hantavirus, 187, 188
Murinae, 124, 125
Musk shrew (*Suncus murinus*),
    123
Mutations, 164–165
  conferring drug resistance, 166
  in hantaviruses, 239–240
Mythology, of Navajo, 43
Myxomatosis, 147–148
Myxoma virus, 147

Nassif, Rogelio, 190
Native American nations, 3
Native Americans
  interviews with, 44–47
  religions of, 42–43
  Sin Nombre HPS among, 35,
    234

Native Americans *(continued)*
  suspicions about U.S.
    government, 17–20
Natural selection, 137
Navajo, 96
  antibody to hantavirus among,
    204
  fear of Chaco Canyon, 48
  forced migration of, 57
  and HLA subtypes, 207
"Navajo Flu," misconception of
    HPS as, 15, 84, 89, 234, 244
Navajo Nation, 42, 43
  increase in population of, 58
Needham, John, 134
Nephropathia epidemica (NE),
    118
  carriers, 119
  in Korea, 120
Neuraminidase, 164, 168
New Mexico, plague in, 9
New York 1 virus, 186, 209
Nichol, Stuart, 33, 240
Nidoko fever, 105
Nuclear weapons testing, 18–19

Oparin, Alexandr Ivanovich, 135
Organ transplantation, and
    immune response, 173
  suppression of, 178
"Outbreak," 216

Padula, Paula, 191
Paraguay, 194–195, 241
Parmenter, Robert, 67–68, 204,
    227
Passive immunization, 217

Pasteur, Louis, 134
Peru current, 50
Petechiae, 103, 194
  of hemorrhagic fever, 86
Peters, C. J., 21, 27, 28, 109, 128,
    215–216
Phlebovirus spp., 111
Phosgene, 10
Pigs, *see* Swine
Piñon mouse (*Peromyscus truei*), 48,
    65
  hantavirus antibodies, 69
Piñon pine, 46, 60, 227
  harvest size and mouse
    population, 47
Plague, 9
Plasmids, 138
Platelets, 211
Polio vaccine, SV40 transmitted by,
    176–177
Polymerase chain reaction (PCR),
    32
Powell, John Wesley, 3
Prairie vole (*Microtus ochrogaster*), 187
Pregnancy, retrovirus-related
    elements and immune
    response, 173–174
Primordial soup, 135
Prodrome, 211
Prospect Hill hantavirus, 126, 187
Proteins, formation of, 137
Public education efforts, 243
Puebloans, ancestral, 56
Puumala virus, 68, 124
  and HLA subtype, 207
  identification, 119
  link to Tula fever, 123
  mortality from, 118
  vaccine against, 219

Rabbit hemorrhagic disease, 157–158

Rabies, recombinant vaccine, 160

Radiation Exposure Compensation Act, 19

Rats
bandicoot (*Bandicota indica*), 123
black (*Rattus rattus*), 113
brown (*Rattus norvegicus*), 31, 113
cotton (*Sigmodon hispidus*), 185
as hantavirus carrier, 112–114
long-tailed pygmy rice (*Oligoryzomys longicaudatus*), 189
rice (*Orysomys palustris*), 185

Redi, Francesco, 134

Reed vole (*Microtus Fortis*), 123

Reoviridae, 171

Retroviruses (Retroviridae), 171
endogenous, 172
RNA to DNA transcription, 172

Reverse transcriptase, 172

Ribavirin, 85
in Rift Valley fever, 155
side effects, 221
Sin Nombre sensitivity to, 220

Ribonucleic acid (RNA), 33, 133, 137
as molecular fossil, 136
in retroviruses, 171–172
segmentation in hantavirus, 239

Rice rat (*Orysomys palustris*), 185

Rift Valley fever, 111, 143, 171
association with El Niño event, 52
as biowarfare agent, 155
mode of transmission, 153
mortality, 154
viral change, 155, 157

Rio Mamore hantavirus, 196

Rodent blooms, 64–65
and Andes HPS, 193
priming of HPS outbreaks, 241–242
reporting of, 65, 66
reversal of, 75–77

Rodents
avoidance of, 222
and debris from, control methods, 228–229
difficulty studying, 74–75
evolution in North America, 125
exposure to, as risk factor, 223–224
hosts of Puumala virus, 71–72
in refugia, hantavirus infection, 246–246

Roseola infantum, 178

Rotaviruses, 171

Russia, Tula fever in, 122–123

Russian flu, 168

Salk, Jonas, 176

Schmaljohn, Connie, 128

Science, 67

Scientific American, 156

Seal plague, of Europe (1988), 178–179

Senate Foreign Operations Subcommittee, 182

Seoul, 112

Seoul hantavirus, 34, 113, 190
spread of, 114–115

Sevilleta National Wildlife Refuge, 63
rodent bloom at, 64–66
Sevilleta (New Mexico), 62
Shalala, Donna, 43
Sickle cell gene, 208
Sigmodontinae, 124, 125
Simian immunodeficiency virus (SIV), 152
Simian virus 40 (SV40), 175
infection in macaque monkey, 176
transmission via polio vaccine, 176–177
Sin Nombre virus, 188
antibody presence
versus HPS, 204–205
testing for, 210
antigenic drift/shift in, 239–240
evolution with rodent hosts, 238
HPS risk from single exposure to, 203–205
identification of, 30–31
incidence in Canada, 197
incubation period, 202
mortality rate, 92
naming of, 94–97
outbreaks beyond Four Corners, 183–184
risk factors for, 223
stability outside of host, 225–226
Slovenia, 121
Smallpox
elimination of, 158–159
vaccine, 160
Snakes, in ecosystem, 47–48
Songo fever, 105
Soviet Union
hantavirus disease in, 104

virus research, 107–108
Spallanzani, Lazzaro, 134
"Spanish" influenza (1918–1920), 10, 25
mortality from, 169
Sverdlovsk (Russia), anthrax outbreak, 155–156
Sweden, hanatvirus in, 71
Swine
and influenza antigenic shift, 168–169
and influenza mutation, 166
in organ transplantation, 175
Symbiosis, 148
Symptoms, hantavirus pulmonary syndrome, 38, 200

Tayinshan disease, 105
Tempest, Bruce, 7, 8
Thailand virus, 123
Thottapalayam virus, 123
Tobetsu virus, 123
Topografov virus, 123
Trade winds, 49–50
Transcription, 133
Translation, 133
Transmission
hantaviruses, 111–112
virus, 141
routes of, 142–143
Transplantation, organ, and immune response, 173
suppression of, 178
Treatment, HPS, protocols, 86–87, 229–231
"Trench nephritis," 102, 120
Trent, William, 18
Tula fever, 122–123

Tula virus, 126
Tuskeegee experiment, 17

United States
    gender and HPV, 235
    HPV fatality rates, 235
    Sin Nombre outbreaks,
        183–184, 236
Uranium mining, 19
U.S. Army Medical Research
        Institute of Infectious
        Diseases, 28, 92, 128, 219
    viral research by, 92–93
U.S. government
    budget cutbacks, 127
    first awareness of hantaviruses,
        100
    overseas disease surveillance by,
        182
    spending on hantavirus
        research, 231–232
    suspicions concerning, 16–18
USAMRIID, see U.S. Army Medical
        Research Institute of
        Infectious Diseases
Ute Tribe, 15

Vaccines, 160, 218–219
    testing problems, 219–220
Vaccinia poxvirus, 160
van Leeuwenhoek, Antoni, 134
The Very Large Mouse Array, 74–75
Vesper mouse (*Calomys laucha*), 194
Virazole, 85
Viruses
    cell entry by, 209
    discovery of, 129
    emerging, 145–146
    in gene therapy, 160–161
    immune response to, 210–213
    mutations of, 141, 144
    origins of, 138–139
    segmented genomes in, 167, 171
    spread of, 141–143
        through medical
            interventions, 174–177
    structure and functions of,
        139–141
    zoonotic, 150–152
"Virus Hunter" (Peters), 21, 216
Virus X theory, 148
Voles
    American meadow (*Microtus
        pennsylvanicus*), 126
    bank (*Clethrionomys glareolus*), 72
    California (*Microtus californicus*),
        187
    European common (*Microtus
        arvalis*), 123
    Japanese (*Clethrionomys
        rufocanus*), 123
    Korean (*Eothenomys regulus*),
        120, 123
    Meadow (*Microtus arvalis*), 31
    population cycles, 71–72
    Prairie (*Microtus ochrogaster*), 187
    reed (*Microtus fortis*), 123

Western harvest mouse
        (*Reithrodontomys megalotis*), 187
Wetherill, Marietta, 47
Whisky, Sergio, 191
White-footed mouse (*Peromyscus
        leucopus*), 65, 186
    in Canada, 197

Whitewater Arroyo virus, 238
Woody, Florena, 6–8, 8, 203
Woody, Franklin, 11, 35, 203
Woody, Jackie, 11–12, 35, 203
World War I, 102
World War II, 122

Xenotransplantation, 174–175, 177

Yellow fever, 143

Yellow-necked field mouse
    (*Apodemus flavicollis*), 121
Yeltsin, Boris, 156
Yersinia pestis, 9
Yugoslavia, 121–122

Zah, Peterson, 43
Zoonoses, 107, 150–152
    introduction by xenotranplant, 174